ATLAS
OF
PARAMEDIC
SKILLS

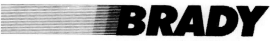

Bryan E. Bledsoe, D.O.
Scott and White Hospital and Clinic
Texas A&M University College of Medicine
Temple, Texas

ATLAS
OF
PARAMEDIC
SKILLS

BRADY
A Prentice Hall Division
Englewood Cliffs, New Jersey 07632

Library of Congress Cataloging in Publication Data

Bledsoe, Bryan E.
    Atlas of paramedic skills.

    Includes bibliographies and index.
1. Medical emergencies—Atlases.   2. Emergency
medical personnel.   I. Title. [DNLM: 1. Allied Health
Personnel—handbooks.   2. Emergency Medicine—atlases.
WB 17 B646a]
RC86.7.B593 1987   616'.025   85-4235
ISBN 0-89303-444-4

Illustration Acknowledgments:
Figures 2.1, 2.25, 2.27—2.29, 2.31—2.33, 2.102—2.115, 3.1, 3.2, 3.10, 4.48—4.51, 4.90, 4.93, 4.97, 5.3, 5.6, 5.8—5.11, 5.14—5.16, 5.18, 5.19, 5.21, 5.22, 5.25, 5.60—5.65, 5.144, 5.145, 5.149—5.153, 6.3, and 6.4 from Charles Phillips, *Paramedic Skills Manual,* © 1980 (A Robert J. Brady Co. publication). Reprinted by permission of Prentice-Hall, Inc., Englewood Cliffs, N.J. Figures 5.7, 5.12, 5.13, 5.23, 5.66, 5.146—148, and 5.154 are also from Phillips, *Paramedic Skills Manual.*

Figures 6.13—6.32 from Gail Walraven, *Basic Arrhythmias,* © 1980 (A Robert J. Brady publication). Reprinted by permission of Prentice-Hall, Inc., Englewood Cliffs, N.J.

Figure 6.54 from L. Meltzer, R. Pinneo, and J. Kitchell, *Intensive Coronary Care: A Manual for Nurses,* 4th ed., © 1983 (A Brady Communications Co., Inc.).

Figures 1.54 and 1.99 and Table 1.4 from E. Rudy and V. Gray, *Handbook of Health Assessment,* © 1981 (Brady Communications Co., Inc.).

Figures 1.45, 1.50, 1.52, 1.56—1.58, 1.88, 1.89, and 1.95—1.97 from D. Langfitt, *Critical Care: Certification preparation and Review,* © 1984 (Brady Communications Co., Inc.).

Figure 5.155 by Z.M. Szalasny, 1983.

© 1987 by Prentice-Hall, Inc.
A Simon & Schuster Company
Englewood Cliffs, New Jersey 07632

Printed in the United States of America

10 9 8 7 6

ISBN 0-89303-444-4   025

Prentice-Hall International (UK) Limited, *London*
Prentice-Hall of Australia Pty. Limited, *Sydney*
Prentice-Hall Canada Inc., *Toronto*
Prentice-Hall Hispanoamericana, S.A., *Mexico*
Prentice-Hall of India Private Limited, *New Delhi*
Prentice-Hall of Japan, Inc., *Tokyo*
Prentice-Hall of Southeast Asia Pte. Ltd., *Singapore*
Editora Prentice-Hall do Brasil, Ltda., *Rio de Janeiro*

DEDICATED TO MY MANY FORMER EMT AND PARAMEDIC STUDENTS WHO ARE AT WORK, IN THE STREETS, DELIVERING EMERGENCY MEDICAL CARE TO THE SICK AND INJURED.

Contents

Preface

Atlas of Paramedic Skills is a complete pictorial guide of the most commonly performed advanced prehospital skills. It is designed as an aid for both EMT-Paramedics and EMT-Intermediates. It thoroughly addresses each of the prehospital skills, briefly describing the skill, its indications, as well as any contraindications or precautions. It then details, step by step, the skill utilizing both photographs and line drawings. At the completion of each skill sequence is a skill check sheet which provides both the instructor and student the criteria for assuring competency. It is important to point out that this textbook is not a substitute for detailed "hands on" instruction under the direction of a qualified instructor. Each of the skills presented must first be practiced on mannequins or fellow students before performing them in a clinical setting. Once in a clinical setting the student should only practice these skills under the direct supervision of a qualified instructor until he or she is determined to be proficient in the particular skill. It is important to point out that many of the skills presented in this book are rarely used even in the more busy Emergency Medical Services systems. Thus it is important that the practicing paramedic review many of these skills periodically. *Atlas of Paramedic Skills* will prove to be an excellent source for routinely reviewing these infrequently used skills.

It is hoped that both the paramedic student as well as the practicing paramedic will find *Atlas of Paramedic Skills* a welcome addition to their personal EMS reference library.

Acknowledgments

The preparation of a book such as *Atlas of Paramedic Skills* is truly a team effort. Without the assistance of the following individuals, this book would certainly not exist.

Thanks must first go to my close friend and supporter Claire Merrick, editor with the Brady Communications Division of Prentice-Hall. With her help, encouragement, and confidence this book finally evolved. Claire inherited this project after the reorganization of Brady in 1985. She was amazingly understanding of my schedule and time constraints as I attended medical school, worked, and prepared this manuscript.

Special thanks also must go to Richard Weimer and David Culverwell, former Brady editors, who asked me to undertake this project and who supported me through the early stages of manuscript production.

The actual writing of a book such as *Atlas of Paramedic Skills* is really the easiest part of the process. The real chore was production of the final project. The big load fell to Alison Gnerre with Prentice-Hall, who took boxes of manuscript, photographs, and illustrations and somehow put it all together into the final product. Alison is a true professional.

Special recognition must go to Brady photographer George Dodson, who photographed over 1,700 pictures for use in this work. He was always eager, interested, and professional. He even found time to show me how to fish the Chesapeake Bay.

Several persons served as models for this text. They include three good natured and professional fire-fighters with the Berwyn Heights, Maryland, Fire Department— Jim Yvorra, David Foust, and James Ward.

Many persons and companies provided technical assistance and supplies for this book. They include James R. Miller with the Prince Georges County, Maryland, Fire Department, who provided much of the equipment utilized in the photographs. The Berwyn Heights Fire Department provided much of the equipment utilized in the photographs. The Berwyn Heights Fire Department provided the ambulance and personnel to operate it. Several of the photographs were shot in the anatomy laboratory at the University of Maryland Medical School. I would like to thank Lou Jordan, director of Prehospital Care with the Maryland Institute of Emergency Medical Services (MIEMS) in Baltimore for setting this up. The actual procedures used in the anatomy lab were performed by David R. Gens, M.D., traumatologist/surgical attendee with MIEMS. He was assisted by Paul J. McCarthy, instructor with the University of Maryland-Baltimore Campus. EMS run reports were generously provided by Chief Bobby Moore, Dallas Fire Department, EMS Division; Bruce Shade, City of Cleveland EMS System; Richard Land, Tennessee Department of Health and Environment, Emergency Medical Services Division; and many others. Special equipment was generously loaned by the Deseret Division of Warner-Lambert; Ohio Medical, Inc.; Count's Rescue Equipment; and Plaza Pharmacy, Fort Worth.

The efforts of my good friends Frank J. Papa, D.O., F.A.C.E.P., and Wayne Schuricht, D.O., F.A.C.E.P. in reviewing the manuscript during various stages of production, are deeply appreciated. In addition, I would like to thank the many national reviewers of this work. Although they remain anonymous, their comments and recommendations are deeply appreciated.

The biggest thanks must go to my patient wife Emma, and my two children, Bryan and Andrea, for their encouragement and support throughout the production of this work as well as my other activities related to emergency medicine and emergency medical services. They make it all worthwhile.

Author's Note

The skills presented in this book are based on national standards. Every effort has been made to assure that they are correct and up to date. It is important to remember that skills procedures vary significantly across the country and from one EMS system to another. If a discrepency is encountered between the procedure presented in this textbook and the procedure preferred by the EMS system medical director, then the paramedic should utilize only those skills approved for use within their respective systems and by the medical director. In addition, many of the skills presented in this textbook may not be utilized by your EMS system. It is the responsibility of the student or practicing paramedic to be familiar with local protocols and procedures.

THE SKILLS PRESENTED IN THIS BOOK ARE ONLY TO BE USED UPON THE DIRECT ORAL OR WRITTEN ORDER OF A LICENSED PHYSICIAN. The importance of complete medical control of prehospital skills, as well as all aspects of prehospital care, cannot be overemphasized.

This text is *not* a substitution for paramedic training. One can only become proficient in the skills described in this book after didactic instruction, laboratory practice, and finally, actual patient practice under the supervision of a certified instructor or licensed physician or nurse.

There are many skills detailed in this text. The presentation of these skills in this text does not constitute a recommendation by the author of those skills, nor does it constitute a recommendation by the author of which skills an EMS system should utilize.

Chapter Objectives

Upon completion of this chapter, the student should be able to:

1. Define the SOAP method of patient assessment.
2. Interview an emergency patient by using open-ended questions followed by focused, closed-ended questions.
3. Use good interview techniques.
4. Understand and use standard questions for interviewing patients with the following:
   - Pain
   - Critical injuries
   - Critical illness
   - Injuries from motor vehicle accidents
   - Burns
   - Lacerations
   - Poisonings and overdoses
5. Complete a primary assessment within the defined time interval.
6. Perform a secondary assessment including assessment of:
   - Level of consciousness
   - Pulse rate and character
   - Respiratory rate and quality
   - Blood pressure
   - The scalp
   - The face
   - The pupils
   - The nose
   - The ears
   - The mouth
   - The neck
   - The chest
   - The upper extremities
   - The abdomen
   - The pelvis and lower extremities
   - The neurological system
7. Understand the indications for and be able to complete an examination of the cranial nerves.
8. Use the Glasgow Coma Scale for evaluation of the patient suffering from a neurological injury or illness.

9. Make a proper assessment of the emergency patient with information gained from both the subjective interview and objective assessment.
10. Formulate a plan on the basis of all of the information gained from the interview, examination, and assessment.
11. Prepare a written report by using accepted local protocols.

1

Advanced Patient Assessment

Assessment of the critically ill or injured patient is the most important of the skills possessed by both the EMT/Intermediate and the EMT/Paramedic. The paramedic acts as the eyes, ears, and hands of the remote base-station physician. Every treatment that follows is dependent upon a thorough and accurate patient evaluation. This chapter will detail the fundamentals of advanced patient assessment as well as provide information on special examination techniques that may be required in special situations.

Before a paramedic can become competent at advanced patient assessment, he or she must be skilled in EMT-level physical assessment. EMT-level assessment is aimed primarily at determining immediate threats to life or limb. Advanced patient assessment, on the other hand, calls for a thorough evaluation of both subjective and objective data to develop an appropriate plan for definitive treatment.

Evaluation of the emergency patient is routinely organized into four distinct components which are collectively referred to as the SOAP system. The term SOAP stands for each of the system's components:

Subjective Data
Objective Data
Assessment
Plan

SUBJECTIVE DATA is that information obtained by interviewing the patient or bystanders. Various feelings expressed by the patient, such as "I have a terrible pain," are considered subjective data because "terrible pain" as described by one individual might be relatively minor; another individual might consider the pain severe.

OBJECTIVE DATA is the information that you learn from the physical examination. Such things as vital signs and other physical findings are considered objective data.

ASSESSMENT is your interpretation of what the subjective and objective findings indicate. In prehospital care, the term assessment should be used rather than diagnosis in describing your impression of the patient's problem. The term diagnosis is reserved for the definitive assessment made by a physician.

The PLAN is simply the treatment that you propose for the patient which takes into consideration the subjective data, objective data, and finally your assessment.

The example in the box illustrates how the SOAP plan applies to a basic emergency situation.

Each patient must be approached in an organized fashion. Jumping to different parts of either the interview or the physical assessment will invariably cause the paramedic to miss pertinent portions of the patient evaluation that may later prove important. The remainder of this chapter will describe the techniques for completing the advanced patient evaluation.

Subjective Data

Subjective data are obtained primarily by interviewing the patient, if conscious, or from bystanders who may have been present when the illness or injury occurred. First responders, who often arrive at the scene before advanced life support units, are an excellent source of subjective data. When interviewing the patient or bystanders, try to gain as much information as possible in as little time as possible. Keeping this in mind, you should word questions in a way such that the patient replies with a maximum amount of information. The best technique for doing this is by using open-ended questions. Open-ended questions allow the patient to describe, in his own words, what his or her problem, or complaint, might be. Once the primary problem is identified, then

---

SOAP Plan Applied to a Basic Emergency Situation

SUBJECTIVE DATA: The patient reports that he fell down several steps as he was leaving a restaurant with some friends. Upon our arrival at the scene he is complaining of severe pain in his right thigh. He denies pain anywhere else. Friends reported that he had "drank a few beers" prior to the accident. The patient has no significant medical history and denies that he is allergic to any medications.

OBJECTIVE DATA: The patient is a 22-year-old, white male with the following vital signs: blood pressure, 110/68; pulse, 110; and respirations, 28. A 2×5 cm bruise is on the right thigh with significant associated swelling. An angulation of the thigh is also noted. Popliteal and pedal pulses are present bilaterally. There appears to be no sensory or motor deficit in the affected leg.

ASSESSMENT: Possible factured right femur.

PLAN: 1.   Administer oxygen at 6-8 L/min.
        2.   Maintain body heat.
        3.   Apply traction splint.
        4.   Administer Lactated Ringer's at 100 mL/h as per physician order.
        5.   Prepare to inflate anti-shock trousers if hypotension ensues.
        6.   Transport to Harris Hospital.

---

close-ended, direct questions may be used to gather any other required information.

Example 1 shows a series of questions that illustrate the advantage of open- over close-ended or direct questions. Although the discussion is hypothetical, it shows that open-ended questions will yield considerably more information in a shorter period of time than standard close-ended, direct questions.

An extremely detailed history is not indicated in the prehospital setting. As soon as the general nature of the patient's problem becomes evident, you should focus your interview on the problem. Specific techniques and guidelines that aid in gathering subjective data from the interview are:

1.   Position yourself close to the patient.
2.   Greet the person by name. This is extremely important. Address children by their first name. All adults should be addressed formally (for example, Mr. Jones). The patient must see that you respect them and they, in turn, will respect you.
3.   Establish and maintain eye contact throughout the interview.
4.   Introduce yourself and tell them with whom you are affiliated (fire department, ambulance service, etc.).
5.   Physical contact, a simple touch, is often very comforting to the patient, especially the elderly.
6.   Keep your questions as open-ended as possible. Once you have asked several open-ended questions, then begin to focus on the patient's problem by using simple closed-ended questions.
7.   Avoid being judgmental. Everyone has a different lifestyle and a different set of moral values.

Keeping these points in mind, you then want to gain specific information

---

EXAMPLE 1.

Close-Ended Questions

Examiner: "Did you fall down the stairs?"
Patient: "Yes."
Examiner: "How did it happen?"
Patient: "I was just coming through the door and tripped."
Examiner: "Did you twist your leg when you fell?"
Patient: "I may have, I can't tell."
Examiner: "Did you try and move after you fell?"
Patient: "No."
Examiner: "Are you in any pain?"
Patient: "Yes, quite a bit of pain."
Examiner: "Where is the pain?"
Patient: "Here, up in my thigh."
Examiner: "Is it a sharp pain?"
Patient: "Yes, pretty sharp."
Examiner: "Is this the only pain you have?"
Patient: "Yes, I think so."

Open-Ended Questions

Examiner: "What happened here?"
Patient: "Well, my buddies and I were leaving the restaurant, and I guess I tripped and fell down the stairs. I'm afraid I broke my leg."
Examiner: "Are you in any pain?"
Patient: "Yes."
Examiner: "Tell me about your pain."
Patient: "Well, it's real sharp, starting here (pointing to thigh) and shoots down my leg. It started hurting right away, in fact, I heard a crack when I fell. It really hurts bad."

---

concerning the injury or illness. Important information includes:

1. The patient's name.
2. The patient's age.
3. Try and determine what is wrong. You should try and distinguish the patient's primary problem and the chief complaint. The chief complaint is the problem that the patient is most concerned about (a psychological factor). The primary problem, on the other hand, is the actual pathophysiological problem (if present). It is essential that you try and get this information from the patient, if conscious. Quite often the chief complaint given by the patient may vary significantly from what bystanders perceive the chief complaint to be.

4. In cases of injury, find out how it happened. In cases of illness, find

out how long the patient has felt ill.

5. Learn if the problem has happened before or if the patient has ever felt this way before.

6. Determine current medical status. Find out if the patient is currently suffering any medical problems that may or may not be related to this episode.

7. Find out what medications are currently being taken.

8. Ask if the patient has any known allergies, especially drug allergies.

After you have gathered general subjective data, then you will want to focus on the patient's immediate problem. Certain information learned during the general interview may warrant further attention. The following questions are examples of complaints or problems that require additional questioning.

Pain

Pain is a subjective symptom, but, it is often the primary concern of the patient. In determining the history of a particular pain, the PQRST format is preferred in the prehospital setting.

P   What PROVOKES the pain? Was the patient doing something that resulted in the pain? What makes the pain better?

Q   What is the QUALITY of the pain? Is it sharp, dull, cutting, throbbing, or crushing?

R   Does the pain RADIATE to any area or is it localized in one spot?

S   What is the SEVERITY of the pain? Is it mild, moderate, severe, or the worst pain the patient has ever experienced?

T   At what TIME did the pain start? Has it gotten progressively worse or somewhat better?

Nausea and Vomiting and/or Diarrhea

- How long (days and hours)?
- How many times in 24 hours?
- Any related pain or injury?
- Any medications taken to relieve it?
- Any blood noted in the vomitus or stools?
- Any change in appetite during the past few days?

Injuries

CRITICALLY INJURED PATIENTS

- What position was the patient in when the injury occurred?
- Where does the patient hurt now?
- Does the patient have any other illnesses?
- Is the patient taking any drugs or medications?
- Does the patient have a bleeding tendency?
- Does the patient have any allergies?
- When was the last meal and fluid intake, and how much?

MOTOR VEHICLE ACCIDENTS

- Where did the accident happen?
- How many cars were involved?
- When did the accident happen?
- Was the patient a driver or passenger?
- What are the injuries and locations?
- Was the patient wearing a seat belt?

BURNS

- Note percent of body area burned.
- Note type of burn (electrical, grease, etc.)
- How, when, and where did the burn occur?

- How long ago?
- What was the environment like?
- How long was the duration of exposure?
- Any treatment so far?

LACERATIONS

- Document location on the body.
- What caused the laceration?
- How long ago?
- Note type of bleeding (arterial, venous, capillary)?
- Is range of motion (ROM) or sensory perception impaired?

POISONINGS AND OVERDOSES

- Note type and amount of material ingested.
- Note time of ingestion.
- Any known reason for ingestion (for example, suicide attempt).
- Note any unusual odors or burns of the mouth.
- Retain any pill bottles.
- Any treatment so far? (Victim may have tried an antidote.)

Once you have gathered an adequate amount of subjective data, objective data should be gathered via the physical assessment. Remember, it should take just a minute or two to gather an adequate amount of subjective data. Try not to interview the patient and perform a physical examination at the same time. Even experienced physicians will only perform the physical exam after completing an adequate history. Remember, the history will clue you in as to what parts of the physical assessment you should pay particular attention to.

Objective Data

The primary method of gathering objective data is by physical examination of the patient. In the emergency setting the physical examination is usually di-

vided into two separate parts. The first part, the PRIMARY ASSESSMENT, is a rapid examination to detect life-threatening problems and includes a rapid evaluation of the airway, breathing, and circulation, and a quick examination for any life-threatening bleeding or significant chest injury. If a problem is noted in the primary assessment, then that problem is treated before proceeding on with the examination.

The second part of the physical assessment, the SECONDARY ASSESSMENT, is a detailed head-to-toe examination. This section will detail the procedures for examining the emergency patient.

The four methods of physical assessment are:

Inspection
Palpation
Percussion
Auscultation

All four methods are not used for every body area. For example, when examining the scalp, only inspection and palpation are necessary. Examination of the chest, on the other hand, requires all four techniques.

When performing a physical examination on a patient it is important to follow the order just presented. Start with inspection, then move to palpation, then, if indicated, finish the examination with percussion and auscultation. The abdomen is a notable exception. Auscultation should precede palpation and percussion because these techniques may affect bowel sounds. However, note that paramedics will rarely, if ever, be called upon to auscultate for the presence of bowel sounds.

Primary Assessment

OVERVIEW   The primary assessment is the first step in the physical examination of any emergency patient. It should include a brief examination of the patient's airway, breathing, circulation, and a quick overview for any signs of severe bleeding or significant chest injury. The primary assessment should not take more than 10-15 seconds to complete.

INDICATIONS Any emergency patient.

CONTRAINDICATIONS None.

PRECAUTIONS Any problems detected during the primary assessment should be treated immediately before proceeding with additional parts of the examination.

REQUIRED EQUIPMENT None.

PROCEDURE As you approach the scene you should quickly assure that the scene is safe (Figure 1.1). If safe, approach and quickly examine the entire

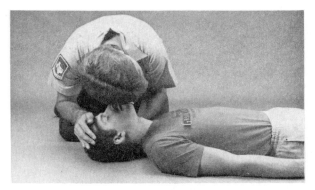

Figure 1.3. Confirm respiration.

patient noting position, location, and appearance. If the patient is conscious, then a brief determination of the mental status may be in order.

Assess the airway (Figure 1.2).

Confirm respiration by noting movement of the chest and passage of an adequate amount of air (Figure 1.3). Note any obvious chest injury (such as a sucking chest wound).

Confirm circulation by palpating the carotid or femoral pulses in unconscious patients or the radial pulses in conscious patients (Figure 1.4).

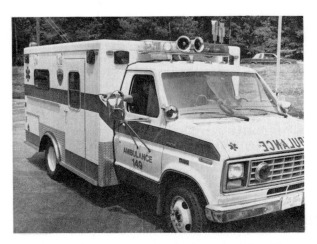

Figure 1.1. Assure that the accident/injury scene is safe.

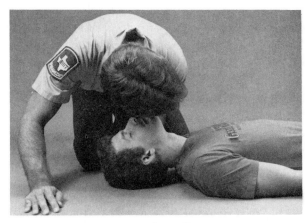

Figure 1.2. Assess the airway.

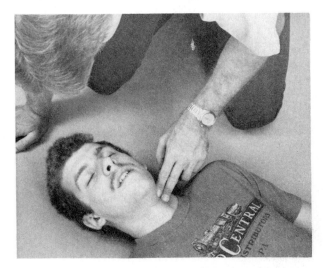

Figure 1.4. Palpate the carotid or femoral pulse to confirm circulation in unconscious patients, or the radial pulse in conscious patients.

As a general rule of thumb, the presence of a radial pulse indicates an approximate systolic pressure of at least 80 mmHg. If absent, the presence of a femoral pulse indicates an approximate systolic pressure of 70 mmHg. If the femoral pulse is absent, then a carotid pulse indicates an approximate systolic pressure of 60 mmHg.

Secondary Assessment

OVERVIEW The secondary assessment includes the patient interview and the physical examination. It is performed only after the primary assessment and correction of any life-threatening situations identified in the primary assessment. The secondary survey includes an evaluation of the vital signs, mental status, and other physical signs and symptoms.

This section will detail the complete secondary assessment of the emergency patient. The secondary assessment should not take more than a few minutes to complete. Obviously, some parts of the secondary assessment are not indicated for every emergency patient. For example, if you were called upon to treat a patient suffering from a gunshot wound to the chest, you would not waste time evaluating such things as motor function. The important consideration in a patient such as this would be to get him to the hospital where he can undergo surgery. Even with advanced life support capabilities there are still cases where the best treatment should be "scoop and run" while attempting advanced life support techniques (for example, IV therapy) enroute.

INDICATIONS Any emergency patient who did not have life-threatening problems discovered in the primary assessment.

PRECAUTIONS The secondary assessment should not take so long that it impedes prompt treatment. Every part of

the secondary assessment may not be indicated for every patient. However, when in doubt, perform the examination.

REQUIRED EQUIPMENT
- Stethoscope
- Sphygmomanometer
- Watch with second hand
- Penlight

OPTIONAL EQUIPMENT
- Reflex hammer
- Tape measure
- Otoscope
- Safety pin

PROCEDURE

Step 1: Determine Level of Consciousness The patient's level of consciousness should be classified (Figure 1.5) according to the following criteria (AVPU):

- Alert—The patient is oriented to person, place, and time.

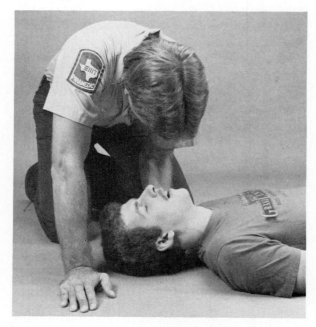

Figure 1.5. Determining the level of consciousness.

- **V**erbal—The patient responds to verbal stimuli.
- **P**ain—The patient responds to painful stimuli. The patient may respond by some attempt to withdraw, moan, or exhibit decorticate or decerebrate posturing.
- **U**nconscious—The patient cannot be aroused.

Step 2: Check Pulse Rate and Character Palpate the radial pulse with the patient's arm near the chest (Figure 1.6) Generally, count the pulse for 15 seconds then multiply by four to obtain the pulse rate. However, in patients with suspected cardiac disease, it might be prudent to count the pulse for a full minute as some dysrhythmias may cause significant variations in the pulse rate. Also note the character of the pulse and classify it as strong or weak, bounding or thready, and regular or irregular. Record your findings on the patient's rec-

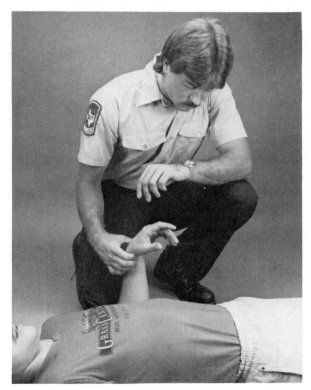

Figure 1.6. Checking pulse rate and character.

ord. Abnormal findings in pulse rate and character are shown in Figure 1.7.

Step 3: Determine Respiratory Rate With your hand still palpating the radial pulse, count the number of respirations in 15 seconds and multiply by four to get the respiratory rate per minute (Figure 1.8). It is important that you make the patient think that you are still taking his pulse so that he will not consciously vary his respiratory pattern. In patients with shallow respirations, it is best to place your hand on the patient's diaphragm (upper aspect of the abdomen) to determine the respiratory rate and pattern. Record your findings on the patient's record. Abnormal findings in respiratory rate are shown in Figure 1.9.

Step 4: Determine Blood Pressure Place the sphygmomanometer firmly on the arm above the elbow (Figure 1.10). Locate the radial pulse. Inflate the cuff until you no longer feel the radial pulse. Note the pressure at which the pulse was lost. This is the approximate systolic pressure (Figure 1.11). Although approximating the systolic pressure is the preferred method, generally, in the emergency setting, this step is usually deleted for the sake of time.

Wait 30 seconds and then inflate the cuff to approximately 20 mmHg above the estimated systolic pressure.

Place the diaphragm of the stethoscope on the brachial artery (Figure 1.12).

Slowly release the pressure and note the point at which the sounds are first heard (systolic) and the point at which the sounds become muffled (first diastolic) and finally when the sounds become absent (second diastolic) (Figure 1.13). Because it is often hard to determine the actual diastolic reading, both diastolic findings should be recorded. Often, you may not be able to distinguish between the first and second diastolic sounds.

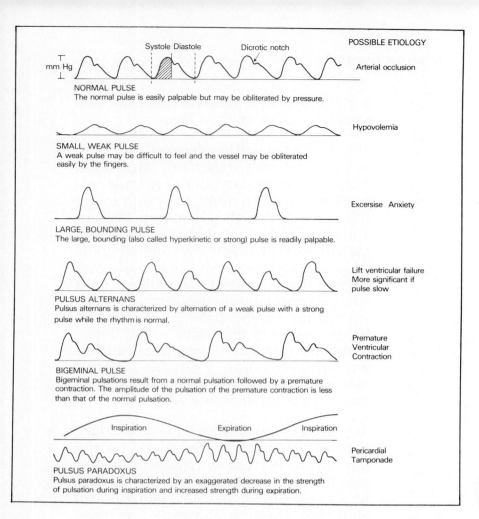

mm Hg

Systole Diastole   Dicrotic notch

POSSIBLE ETIOLOGY

Arterial occlusion

NORMAL PULSE
The normal pulse is easily palpable but may be obliterated by pressure.

Hypovolemia

SMALL, WEAK PULSE
A weak pulse may be difficult to feel and the vessel may be obliterated easily by the fingers.

Excersise Anxiety

LARGE, BOUNDING PULSE
The large, bounding (also called hyperkinetic or strong) pulse is readily palpable.

Lift ventricular failure
More significant if pulse slow

PULSUS ALTERNANS
Pulsus alternans is characterized by alternation of a weak pulse with a strong pulse while the rhythm is normal.

Premature Ventricular Contraction

BIGEMINAL PULSE
Bigeminal pulsations result from a normal pulsation followed by a premature contraction. The amplitude of the pulsation of the premature contraction is less than that of the normal pulsation.

Inspiration   Expiration   Inspiration

Pericardial Tamponade

PULSUS PARADOXUS
Pulsus paradoxus is characterized by an exaggerated decrease in the strength of pulsation during inspiration and increased strength during expiration.

Figure 1.7. Abnormal findings in pulse rate and character.

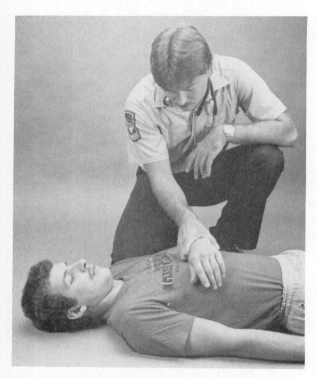

Figure 1.8. Determining respiratory rate.

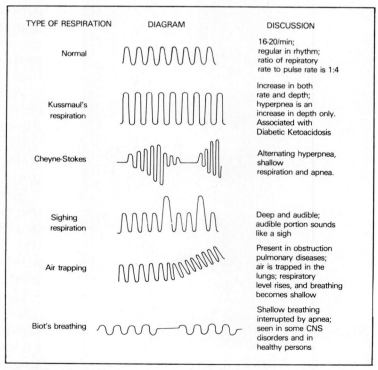

TYPE OF RESPIRATION	DIAGRAM	DISCUSSION
Normal		16-20/min; regular in rhythm; ratio of repiratory rate to pulse rate is 1:4
Kussmaul's respiration		Increase in both rate and depth; hyperpnea is an increase in depth only. Associated with Diabetic Ketoacidosis
Cheyne-Stokes		Alternating hyperpnea, shallow respiration and apnea.
Sighing respiration		Deep and audible; audible portion sounds like a sigh
Air trapping		Present in obstruction pulmonary diseases; air is trapped in the lungs; respiratory level rises, and breathing becomes shallow
Biot's breathing		Shallow breathing interrupted by apnea; seen in some CNS disorders and in healthy persons

Figure 1.9. Abnormal findings in respiratory rate.

10

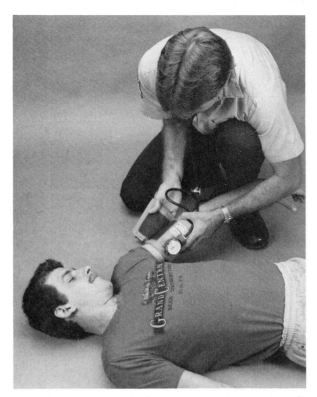

Figure 1.10. Place sphygmomanometer firmly on the arm above the elbow.

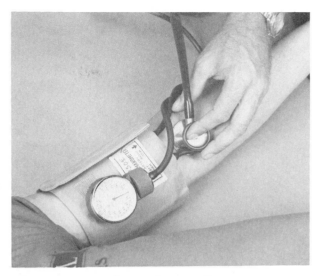

Figure 1.12. Place the stethoscope over the brachial artery.

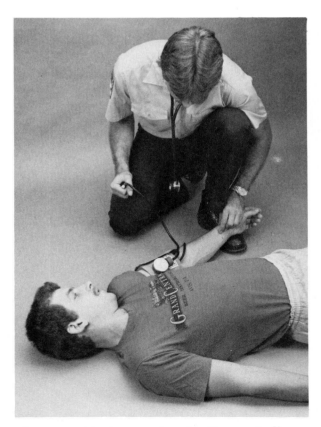

Figure 1.11. Approximate the systolic pressure.

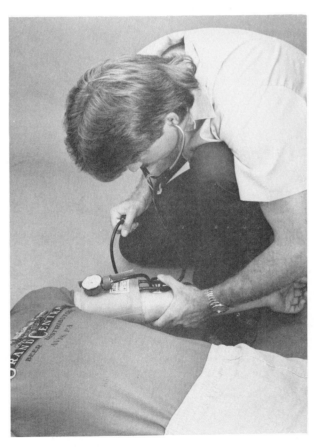

Figure 1.13. Determine the blood pressure.

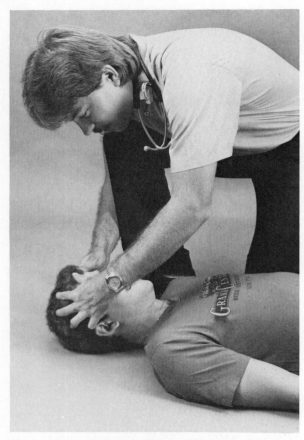

Figure 1.14. Inspection and palpation of the scalp.

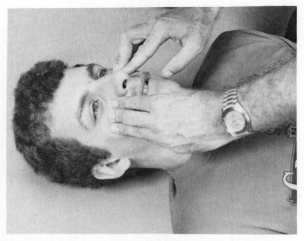

Figure 1.15. Examination of the face and facial bones.

Abnormal findings upon facial examination include:

1. Battle's sign (Figure 1.16), a bruising over the mastoid area, is often seen in fractures of the basilar skull.
2. Raccoon's eyes (Figure 1.17), a bilateral bruising of the periorbital area, is also associated with basilar skull fractures.

Step 5: Examination of the Scalp INSPECT the scalp for any lacerations, bleeding, or bruising (Figure 1.14) Note the presence of hair and any foreign materials or parasites that might be present (such as glass from a shattered windshield).

PALPATE the scalp noting any deformity of the skull. Pay particular attention to any swelling and note its location and size.

Step 6: Examination of the Face INSPECT the face for obvious lacerations, asymmetry, bruising, or other discolorations (Figure 1.15). Pay particular attention to the mastoid area (behind the ear) and the area around the eyes.

PALPATE the facial bones again, and note symmetry or tenderness.

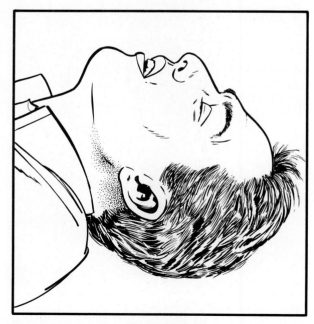

Figure 1.16. Battle's sign.

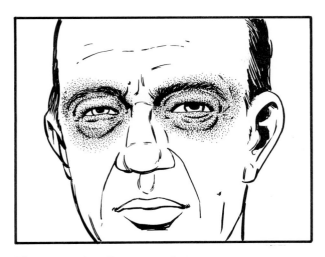

Figure 1.17. Raccoon's eyes.

3. Temporomandibular dislocations (Figure 1.18) occur when the mandible slips from its socket in the temporal bone. This usually occurs when a patient opens his or her mouth extremely wide.

Step 7: Examination of the Pupils IN-SPECT the pupils carefully by comparing one eye to the other (Figure 1.19). Note the SIZE of the pupils and whether or not they are equal. Note the SHAPE of the pupil. They should normally be round.

Note the direct REACTION of the pupil to light (Figure 1.20). The pupil

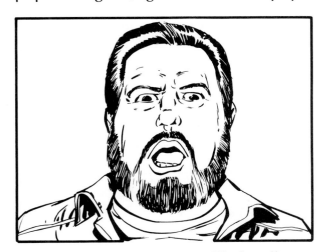

Figure 1.18. Temporomandibular dislocation.

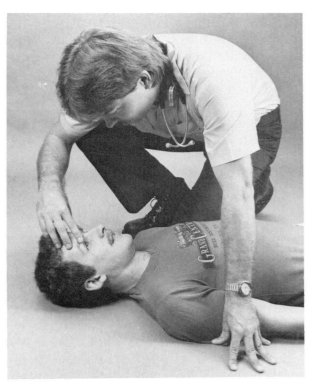

Figure 1.19. Inspect the pupils noting equality and shape.

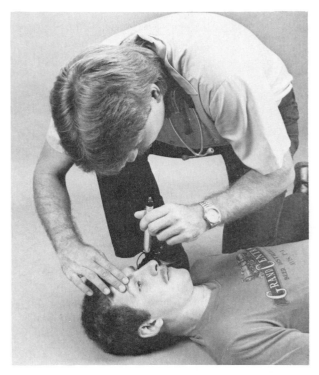

Figure 1.20. Inspect the direct pupillary reaction.

should immediately constrict when a penlight is directed into the eye. Normally both eyes constrict when a penlight is shown in one eye.

When testing pupillary reflexes note both the direct and indirect (opposite eye) reaction (Figure 1.21). This is known as a consensual response.

Finally, test for accommodation (Figure 1.22). Place your finger about 12 inches from the patient's nose and ask him to follow it with his eyes as you move it toward his nose. Normally, the pupils will constrict as your finger approaches the nose. This is referred to as accommodation.

NOTE: Determine whether or not the patient has an artificial eye or has recently received medication such as mydriatics (drugs used to dilate the eyes) which may affect pupil size. Also, some patients will have a pupillary abnormal-

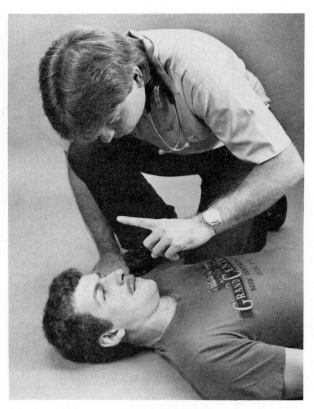

Figure 1.22. Test for accommodation.

ity that has been present for some time and generally is not cause for alarm.

The result of the pupillary exam is normally recorded as PERRLA meaning the pupils are equal, round, and reactive to light and accommodation.

Inequality of the pupils is referred to as ANISCORIA and is often seen in cases of brain damage (Figure 1.23). It is important to note that some aniscoria is present in a good percentage of the population.

Dilated, nonreactive pupils (Figure 1.24) are associated with severe brain hy-

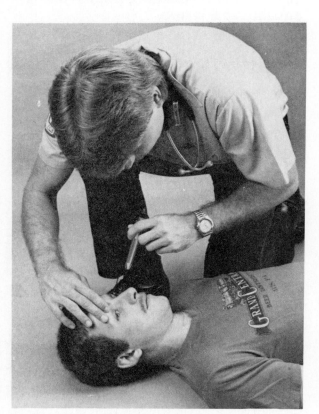

Figure 1.21. Note the indirect pupillary reaction.

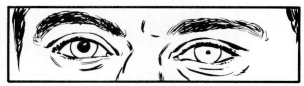

Figure 1.23. Aniscoria—Inequality of the pupils.

poxia and with certain drugs such as atropine.

Very small, equal pupils (Figure 1.25) are often associated with narcotic usage.

Argyll-Robertson pupils are small, irregular pupils that react to accommodation but not to light (Figure 1.26). They are often, but not necessarily, related to tertiary syphilis (tabes dorsalis).

Oculomotor nerve paralysis is characterized by a dilated pupil that neither reacts to light or accommodation (Figure 1.27). Deviation of the eye laterally and downward may also be present.

Step 8: Examination of the Nose IN-SPECT the nose for symmetry and deformity.

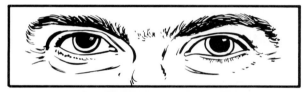

Figure 1.24. Dilated, nonreactive pupils.

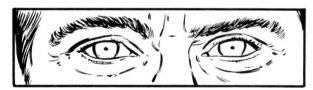

Figure 1.25. Small, equal pupils.

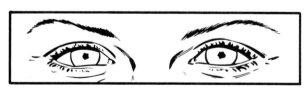

Figure 1.26. Argyll-Robertson pupils.

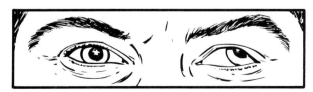

Figure 1.27. Oculomotor nerve paralysis.

Also note any bleeding or the presence of blood-tinged, clear fluid (Figure 1.28).

Clear, watery (often blood-tinged) discharge accompanying a head injury is often indicative of a skull fracture (Figure 1.29).

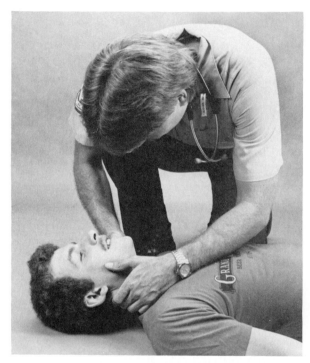

Figure 1.28. Inspect the nose noting especially fluid discharge.

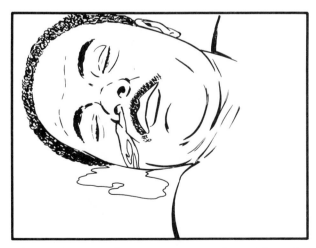

Figure 1.29. Clear, watery (often blood-tinged) discharge is often indicative of a skull fracture.

PALPATE the nose for symmetry and tenderness. Test the patency of the nostrils by compressing one nostril lightly and asking the patient to breathe through the other nostril. Repeat for the opposite nostril.

In addition to the presence of blood-tinged, clear fluid, other abnormal findings include:

1. Anterior epistaxis—commonly associated with blows to the nose. The blood primarily flows through the nostrils (Figure 1.30).
2. Posterior epistaxis (Figure 1.31)—associated with hypertension and occurs more frequently in the elderly. Blood primarily drains into the throat.

Step 9: Examination of the Ears INSPECT the external ear for lacerations. Inspect the external auditory canal for blood or clear watery fluid (Figure 1.32). The presence of watery fluid may indicate a skull fracture. The presence of blood may indicate damage to the middle or inner ear. Make sure that any bleeding is not from a nearby scalp laceration before deciding that the source of the bleeding is indeed the ear. Note also the mastoid area if missed during the earlier portion of examination.

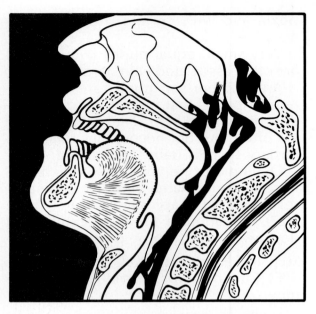

Figure 1.31. Posterior epistaxis where blood flow primarily drains into the throat.

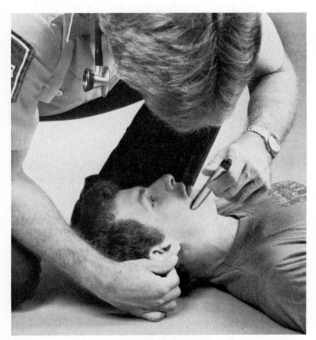

Figure 1.32. Inspect the ear for blood or clear watery fluid.

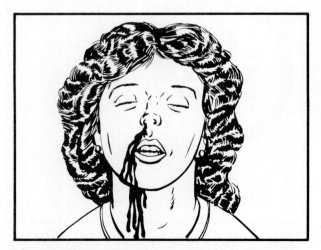

Figure 1.30. Anterior epistaxis where blood flow is through the nostrils.

Step 10: Examination of the Mouth INSPECT the mouth first noting any foreign bodies or fractured teeth in the oropharynx (Figure 1.33). Note es-

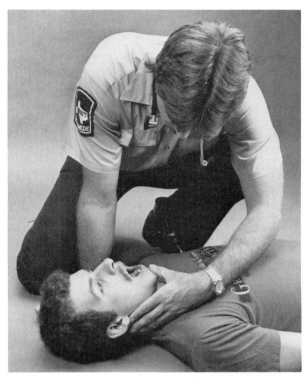

Figure 1.33. Examine the mouth and oral cavity for loose teeth, lacerations, and for perioral cyanosis.

pecially any oral lacerations or lesions that may be bleeding and can, conceivably, occlude the airway. Note any cyanosis present in the perioral area. This is an important place to examine for cyanosis in dark-skinned individuals.

Step 11: Examination of the Neck IN-SPECT the neck for any obvious trauma or bruising (Figure 1.34). Expose the entire neck and note if a stoma is present.

Observe the neck during respirations and note especially suprasternal retraction and hypertrophy of the accessory respiratory muscles (Figure 1.35).

PALPATE the neck beginning superiorily. Follow the trachea down (Figure 1.36) noting any deviation. Assume that a C-spine injury might exist and avoid moving the neck at all. If tracheal deviation is suspected, mark the location of the trachea with a ball-point pen for comparison later.

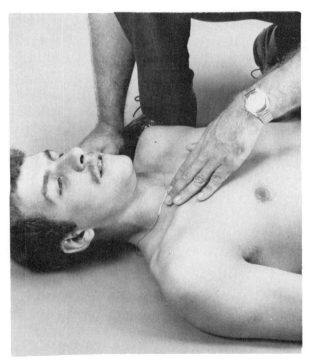

Figure 1.34. Inspect the neck for bruising or trauma.

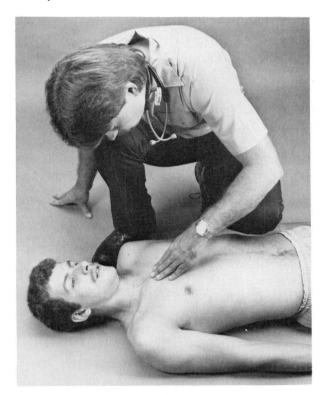

Figure 1.35. Note any suprasternal retraction and inspect for developed accessory muscles.

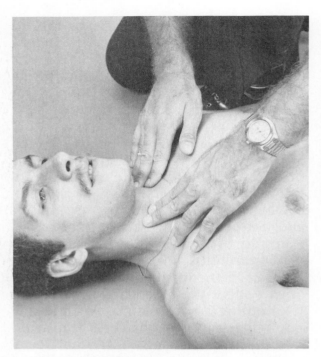

Figure 1.36. Palpate the trachea noting any deviation.

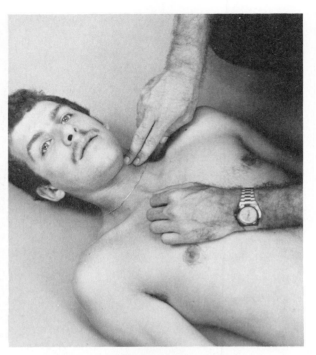

Figure 1.37. Palpate the carotid pulses individually.

Palpate the carotid pulses *individually*, and note rate and character (Figure 1.37). Check for neck vein distension and filling.

Gently palpate the cervical spine noting any deformity or tenderness (Figure 1.38). After you remove your hands from under the patient's neck be sure to check for the presence of blood.

Note any jugular venous distension with the patient at approximately 45° (Figure 1.39).

AUSCULTATE the carotid arteries with the bell of the stethoscope for bruits or thrills (Figure 1.40). A bruit is a blowing sound, and a thrill is an actual vibration. Both sounds are associated with turbulent blood flow through the artery.

Abnormal findings and conditions include:

1. Tracheal deviation occurs with tension pneumothorax (Figure 1.41). The trachea will normally deviate away from the side of the injury.

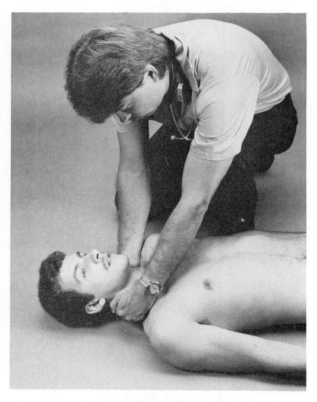

Figure 1.38. Gently palpate the cervical spine noting any deformity or tenderness.

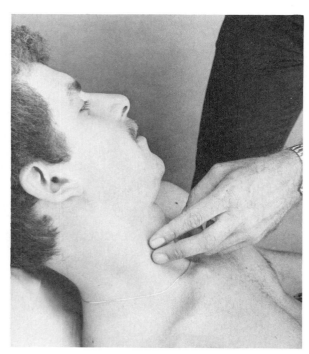

Figure 1.39. Any jugular venous distension with the patient at approximately 45°.

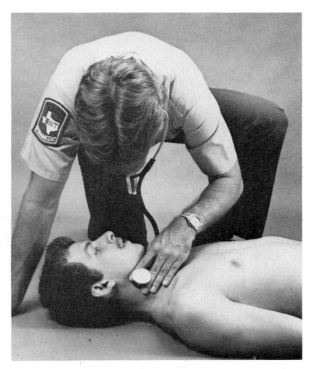

Figure 1.40. Auscultate the carotid arteries with the bell of the stethoscope noting any bruits or thrills.

2. Patients with chronic obstructive pulmonary disease tend to have well-developed accessory muscles and often have suprasternal retraction (Figure 1.42).

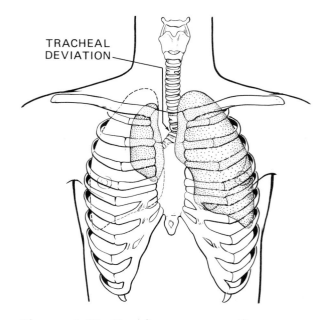

TRACHEAL DEVIATION

Figure 1.41. Tension pneumothorax.

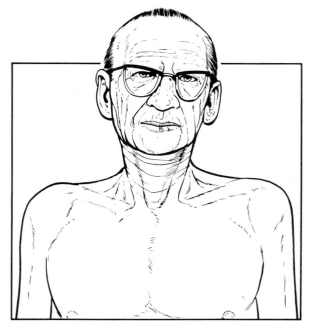

Figure 1.42. Well-developed accessory muscles and suprasternal retraction.

3. Jugular venous distension (Figure 1.43) is associated with such things as cardiogenic shock, pericardial tamponade, tension pneumothorax, traumatic asphyxia, and right heart failure.

Step 12: Examination of the Chest   INSPECT the chest for symmetry and respiratory pattern (Figure 1.44). Note any

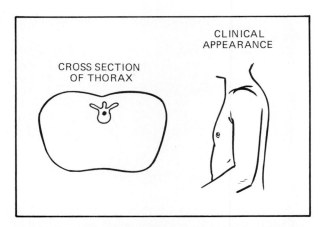

Figure 1.45. Appearance of the normal adult chest.

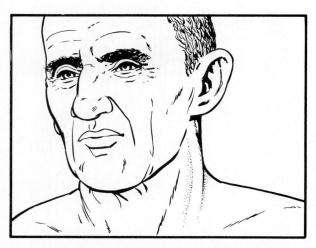

Figure 1.43. Jugular venous distension.

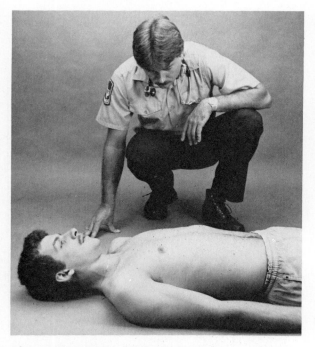

Figure 1.44. Inspect the chest wall for symmetry and respiratory pattern.

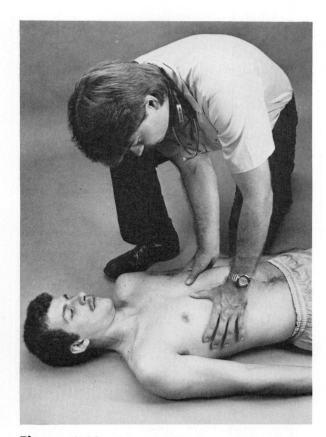

Figure 1.46.

areas of paradoxical breathing. Note general structure and configuration of chest wall (Figure 1.45).

PALPATE the entire chest noting any tenderness, crepitus (don't elicit!), or subcutaneous emphysema (Figure 1.46).

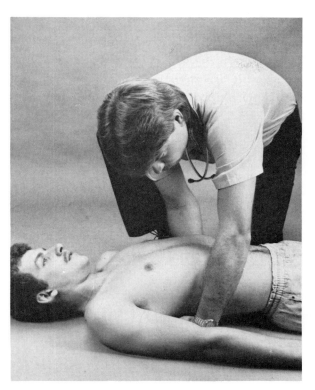

Figure 1.47.

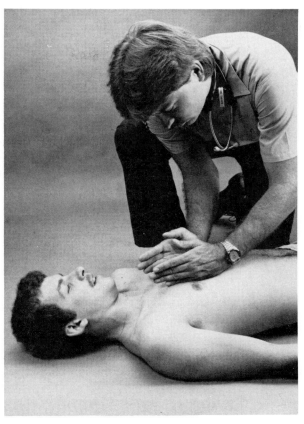

Figure 1.49.

Palpate the posterior chest and thoracic spine (Figure 1.47). Note any deformities. Be sure to inspect your hands for any signs of bleeding after palpating the posterior chest (Figure 1.48). If the patient is complaining of respiratory distress you might also evaluate tactile fremitus (Figure 1.49). Tactile fremitus is the vibration felt in the chest during speaking. Ask the patient to say ninety-nine while you feel for vibration (Figure 1.50). See Table 1.1 for characteristics of tactile fremitus. It should be evaluated by comparing symmetrical areas of the chest. Evaluation of tactile fremitus is of little use in the prehospital setting.

Evaluate the chest by PERCUSSION comparing symmetrical areas (Figures 1.51 and 1.52).

Use of percussion is generally limited to suspected cases of pneumothorax or pulmonary edema.

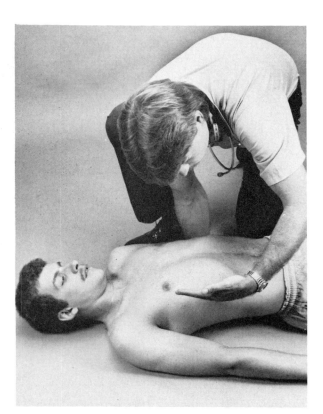

Figure 1.48.

Table 1.1.   Characteristics of Tactile Fremitus.

Type of Fremitus	Characteristics
Increased vocal fremitus	Increased vocal fremitus occurs in pneumonia, compressed lung, or pulmonary fibrosis. Solid medium conducts sound better than porous.
Decreased or absent tactile fremitus	Occurs in pneumothorax and emphysema.
Pleural friction rub	Occurs when inflamed pleural surfaces rub together. It is felt as a grating.
Rhoncal fremitus	Coarse vibrations produced by passage of air through mucous in larger airways.

Table 1.2.   Description of Types of Percussion.

Note	Intensity	Pitch	Quality	Normal Location
Flat	Soft	High	Quite dull	Thigh
Dull	Soft	Medium	Thudlike	Liver
Resonant	Moderate	Low	Hollow	Lung
Hyperesonant	Very Loud	Lower	Booming	Emphysema
Tympanic	Loud	High	Musical	Stomach

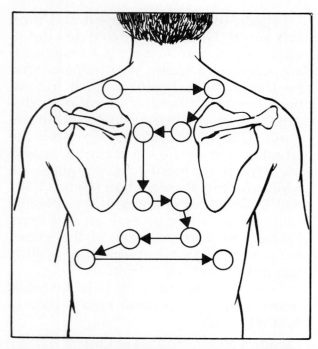

Figure 1.50. Pattern for assessing tactile fremitus.

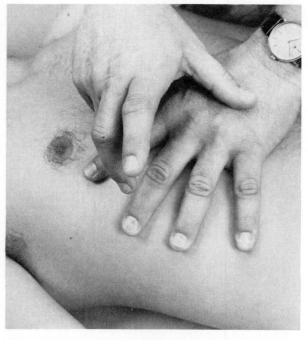

Figure 1.51. Percuss the entire chest using the technique shown.

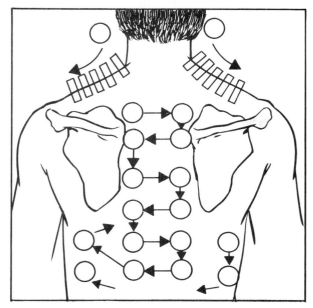

Figure 1.52. Pattern for percussion of the chest comparing symmetrical areas.

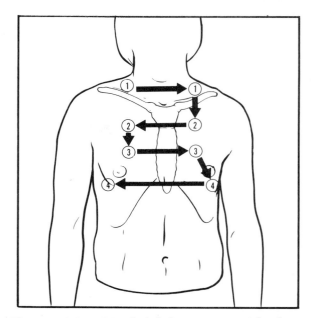

Figure 1.54. Method for symmetrical auscultation of the chest.

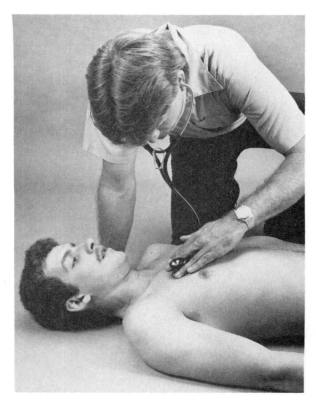

Figure 1.53. Auscultate the chest using the diaphragm of the stethoscope.

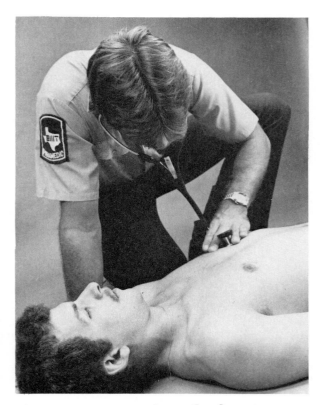

Figure 1.55. Auscultate the heart.

AUSCULTATE the entire chest using the diaphragm of the stethoscope (Figure 1.53).

Once again, compare symmetrical areas (Figure 1.54). Listen to the breath sounds and note their intensity and any variations from normal. Abnormal breath sounds and their causes are shown in Table 1.3.

AUSCULTATE the heart, and note the rate, rhythm, and any obvious murmur (Figure 1.55).

Table 1.3. Types of Abnormal Breath Sounds.

Sound	Cause	Description
Rales—fine to medium	Air passing through liquid in small air passages and alveoli	Noncontinuous crackling sounds. (To simulate, rub a few hairs together over your ear.) Heard at end of inspiration, over the peripheral lung. If widespread, usually indicates pneumonia. Also found in congestive heart failure.
Rales—medium to coarse (coarse are somtimes called *rhonchi*)	Air passing through liquid in the bronchioles, bronchi, and trachea	Louder than fine rales. Usually heard on late inspiration or expiration over airways. Heard in bronchitis, bronchiectasis, resolving pneumonia, emphysema, pleural effusion, and congestive heart failure.
Rhonchi-sibilant (wheeze)	Air passing through wet and swollen airways	Continuous high-pitched wheezy or squeaky sounds heard over the airways, more pronounced during exhalation. Usually found in patients with asthma and chronic obstructive pulmonary disease. *Caution*: Absence of wheeze in asthmatic patient may indicate acute bronchospasm with severely restricted air flow.
Rhonchi-sonorous	Same as for sibilant	Continous low-pitched moaning or snoring sounds. May clear with coughing. Heard mainly during exhalation. Indicates secretions or obstructive masses in the larger airways.
Friction rub	Rubbing together of inflamed and irritated pleural surfaces	Grating or creaking sounds. Heard during both inspiration and exhalation. Cough has no effect. Found in patients with pleurisy, TB, pulmonary infarction, pneumonia, or lung cancer.

Abnormal findings are as follows:

1. Barrel chest is associated with emphysema and is due to development of the accessory respiratory muscles (Figure 1.56).
2. Funnel chest (pectus excavatum) is characterized by compression of the lower part of the sternum (Figure 1.57).
3. Pigeon chest (pectus carinatum) is characterized by an anteriorly displaced sternum (Figure 1.58).

Special Note:

It is often important, both in the written and radio report, to describe the location of various wounds or lesions involving the chest. The following method for ANATOMICAL DESCRIPTION OF CHEST WOUNDS OR LESIONS is frequently used (Figures 1.59–1.61).

Step 13: Exmination of the Upper Extremities INSPECT the upper extremities for symmetry, deformity, and any obvious injuries beginning at the

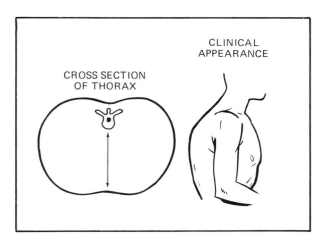

Figure 1.56. Barrel chest.

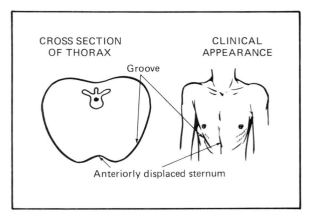

Figure 1.58. Pigeon chest.

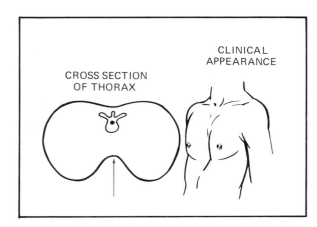

Figure 1.57. Funnel chest.

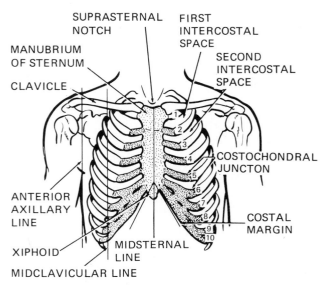

Figure 1.59. Topographical anatomy of the chest (front view).

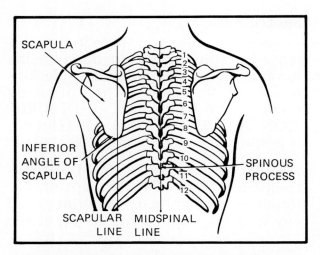

Figure 1.60. Topographical anatomy of the chest (back view).

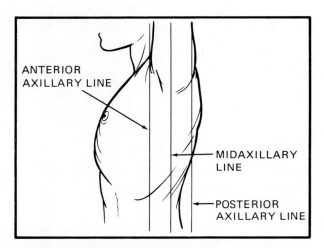

Figure 1.61. Topographical anatomy of the chest (side view).

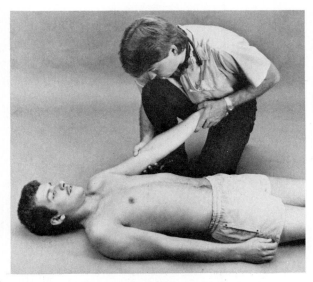

Figure 1.62. Inspect the upper extremities for symmetry and deformity.

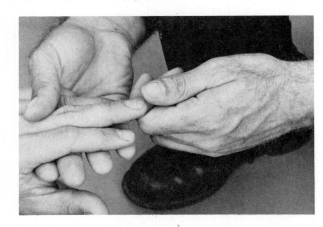

Figure 1.63. Inspect the fingernail beds and finger tips.

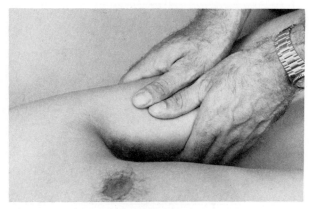

Figure 1.64. Palpate the upper extremities.

shoulder and proceeding down the arms (Figure 1.62). Inspect the hands paying particular attention to the fingernail beds and the shapes of the fingers themselves (Figure 1.63). Table 1.4 shows abnormalities or variations of nails.

PALPATE the upper extremities (Figure 1.64) beginning at the shoulder and proceeding down the arm. Note any tenderness or deformity.

Palpate the brachial (Figure 1.65) and radial (Figure 1.66) pulses bilaterally.

Table 1.4. Abnormalities or Variations of Nails.

Abnormality or Variation	Cause	Figure
Badly mutilated, bitten	Usually nervous habit of biting	
Beau's line	Matrix forms transverse indentation during severe illness	
Clubbing: early, late	Often associated with cardiac or respiratory disorders	EARLY LATE
Splinter hemorrhages	Thin, brownish, flame-shaped lines in the nail bed. Occurs with minor trauma, emboli from subacute bacterial endocarditis or without specific cause	
Red half-moons in nail bed	Cardiac failure	
Subungual hematoma	Blow to nail	
Subungual glomus tumor	Growth under nail	
Paronychia	Inflamed skin around nail	

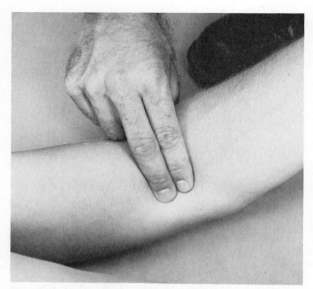

Figure 1.65. Palpate the brachial pulses.

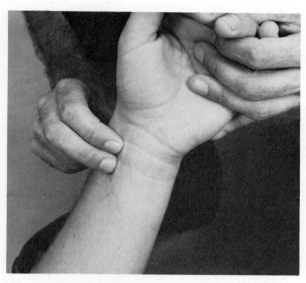

Figure 1.66. Palpate the radial pulses.

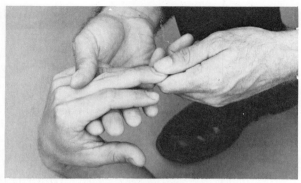

Figure 1.67. Note capillary refill by compressing the fingernail and noting return of coloration. Coloration should return within 1 to 2 seconds.

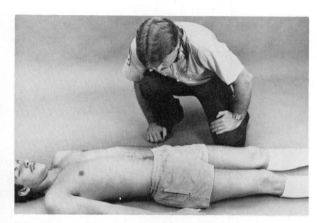

Figure 1.68. Inspect the abdomen for distension, bruising, lacerations, or eviscerations.

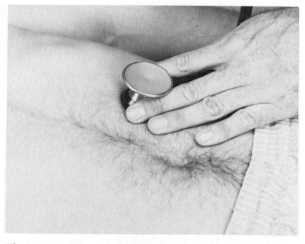

Figure 1.69. Auscultate the abdomen for the presence of bowel sounds.

Palpate the hands. Compress the fingernail bed and note capillary refill (Figure 1.67). Ask the patient to move his fingers. Test grip strength bilaterally.

Step 14: Examination of the Abdomen   INSPECT the abdomen noting any distension, bruising, wounds, or evisceration (Figure 1.68).

AUSCULTATE all four abdominal quadrants for the presence of bowel sounds (Figure 1.69). The absence of bowel sounds is considered pathological. However, in order to state that bowel sounds are absent, you must auscultate for at least five minutes. This often makes auscultation of bowel sounds in the prehospital care of questionable value and generally should never be performed. It is included here merely as a point of interest.

PALPATE the abdomen. If the patient has abdominal pain you should leave the quadrant where the pain is located until the end of the examination so as to avoid guarding (Figure 1.70).

Palpate superficially, then, if time permits, palpate deeper structures (Figure 1.71). Note any areas of tenderness or guarding.

Palpate the lower back and lumbar spine noting any tenderness or deformity (Figure 1.72). Inspect the palms of your hands for the presence of blood.

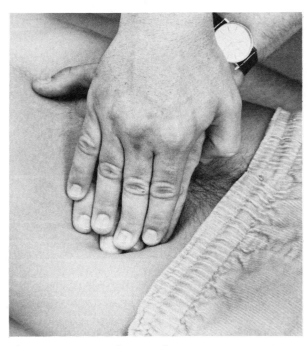

Figure 1.71. Palpate deeper structures noting tenderness or guarding.

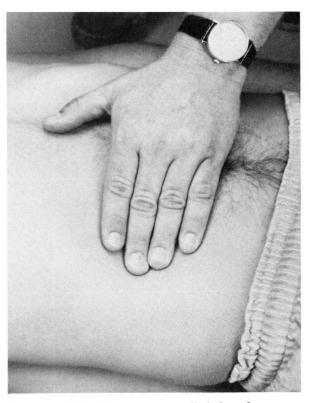

Figure 1.70. Begin superficial palpation; avoid areas where the patient reports pain.

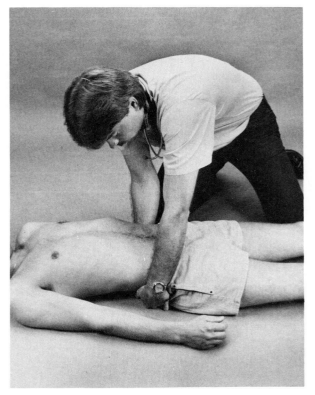

Figure 1.72. Palpate the lower back and lumbar spine.

Step 15: Examination of the Pelvis and Lower Extremities INSPECT the lower extremities and note symmetry, obvious deformities, and any injuries (Figure 1.73). Begin at the pelvis, and proceed toward the feet.

Inspect the toes for gangrene and/or tissue necrosis (Figure 1.74).

Palpate the lower extremities beginning first at the pelvis and proceeding down the leg. Note any tenderness or deformity (Figures 1.75 and 1.76).

Palpate the femoral pulses for equality (Figure 1.77).

Palpate the thigh (Figure 1.78). Compare the diameter of each thigh. If swelling is present, or if a femoral fracture is suspected, measure the circumference of the thigh with a cloth tape measure if time permits. This measurement will aid the emergency department personnel in estimating the amount and magnitude of bleeding into the thigh.

Compress the pre-tibial area and the calves and note any swelling or pain (Figure 1.79). Pain in this area may be indica-

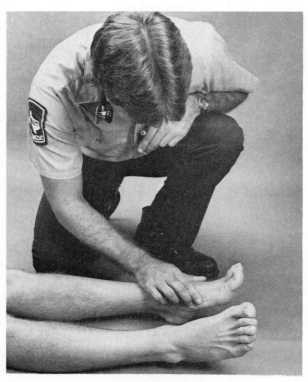

Figure 1.74. Inspect the toes for tissue necrosis or gangrene.

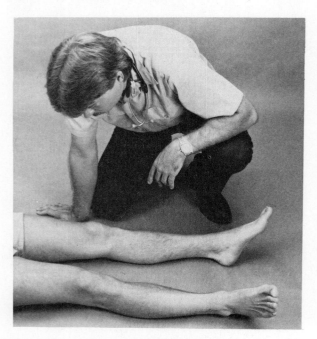

Figure 1.73. Inspect the lower extremities and note symmetry and any obvious deformities or injuries.

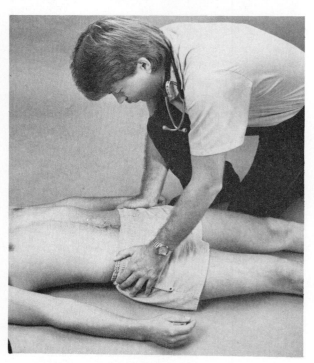

Figure 1.75. Palpate the pelvis.

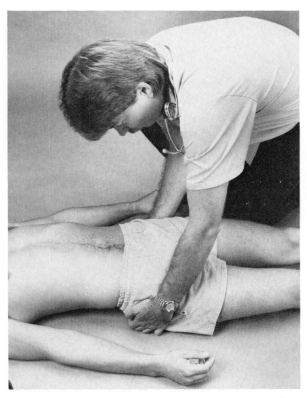

Figure 1.76. Compress the pelvis at the iliac crests and note any tenderness.

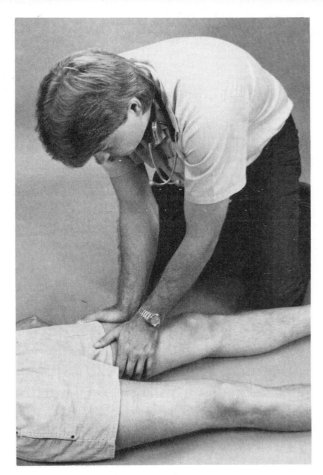

Figure 1.78. Palpate the thigh.

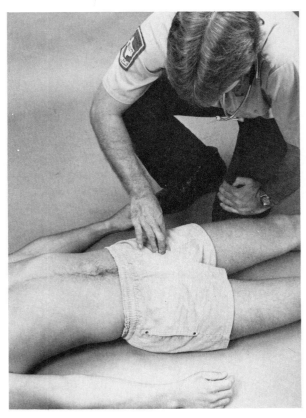

Figure 1.77. Palpate the femoral pulses.

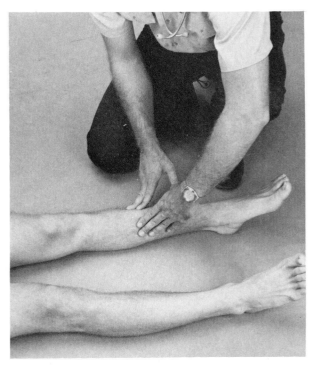

Figure 1.79. Compress the pre-tibial area and the calves.

tive of a compartment syndrome or deep venous thrombosis.

Palpate for edema in both ankles (Figure 1.80). Flex the foot, and note whether or not this causes any pain in the patient's calf. If pain occurs, this pain is referred to as "Homan's Sign" and indicates the possible presence of deep venous thrombosis. This test may aid in the diagnosis of such disorders as pulmonary embolism.

Evaluate the pedal pulses bilaterally (Figure 1.81).

Have the patient wiggle both feet to evaluate motor function (Figure 1.82).

Step 16: Examination of the Neurological System   Evaluation of the neurological system is an important part of the physical examination. It includes evaluation of the mental status, reflexes, and both motor and sensory functions. Remember, a complete evaluation of the nervous system is not indicated in every

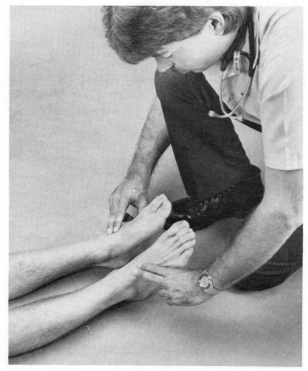

Figure 1.81. Evaluate the pedal pulses bilaterally.

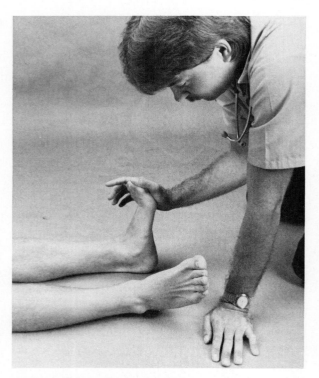

Figure 1.80. Flex the foot.

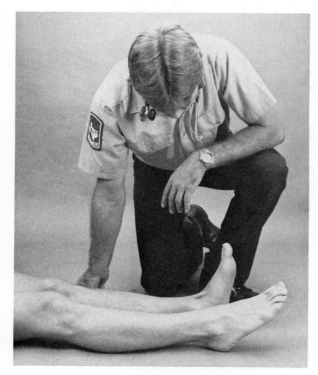

Figure 1.82. Have the patient wiggle both feet.

patient and should not be a reason for delaying transport.

The MENTAL STATUS is evaluated by asking the patient a series of questions (Figure 1.83). The questions are designed to determine the patient's orientation to person, place, and time. Commonly used questions include:

1. What is your name? (Person)
2. Where are you? (Place)
3. What day is this? (Time)
4. About what time of day is it? (Time)

If you are unsure if the patient's responses are appropriate, ask additional questions such as:

1. Who is the president of the United States?
2. What city do you live in?
3. What is your address?
4. How old are you?

Sometimes it may be appropriate to ask nonsense questions to see if the pa-

tient is fully oriented. Some of the more popular nonsense questions are:

1. How many nickles in a week?
2. Do helicopters eat their young?

A patient who is totally oriented to person, place, and time should be able to give appropriate responses to all of the questions just listed.

Test the REFLEXES by striking the appropriate tendon with a reflex hammer or your fingers. The only deep tendon reflexes that should be tested in the prehospital setting are the brachial (Figure 1.84) and the patellar (Figure 1.85) reflexes. Routine examination of the deep tendon reflexes is rarely indicated in prehospital assessment.

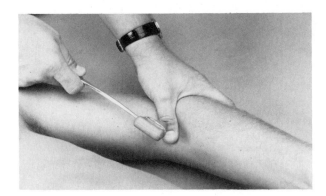

Figure 1.84. Test the brachial reflexes by comparing both arms.

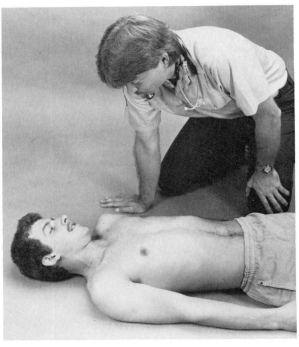

Figure 1.83. Evaluate the mental status.

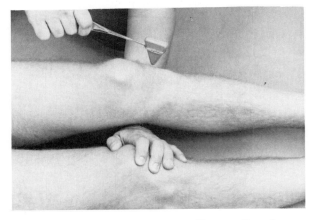

Figure 1.85. Test the patellar reflex by comparing both legs.

When indicated (for example, in head or spine injuries), the paramedic should also evaluate the Babinski reflex (Figure 1.86) and withdrawal to pain (Figure 1.87). Figure 1.88 shows a negative

Babinski reflex (which is considered a normal finding). A positive Babinski reflex (Figure 1.89) is normal in children from 1 to 2 years of age. Otherwise, positive Babinski reflex is indicative of a

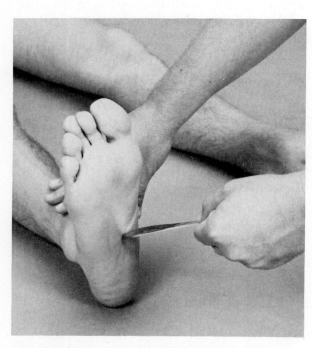

Figure 1.86. Test the Babinski reflex.

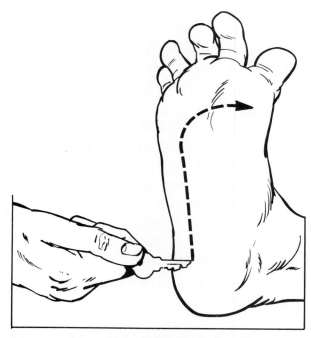

Figure 1.88. Positive Babinski reflex (considered pathological).

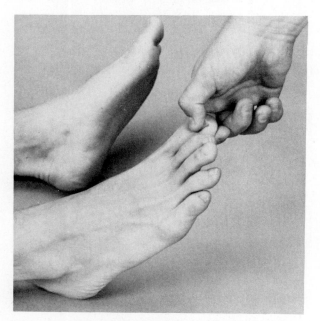

Figure 1.87. Test withdrawal to pain by pressing firmly on the nail beds.

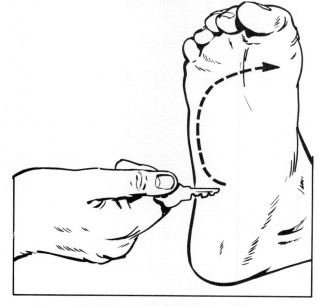

Figure 1.89. Negative Babinski reflex.

disorder of the pyramidal tracts (motor function).

Finally, evaluate sensory and motor function to the extremities (Figure 1.90–1.93), especially if you suspect neurological injury.

Then, note the general appearance of the patient (Figure 1.94). Also note any

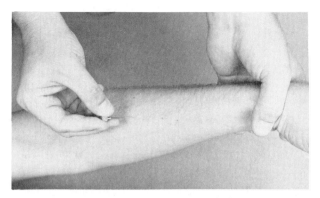

Figure 1.92. Test sensory function in the upper extremity by asking the patient to identify sharp or dull.

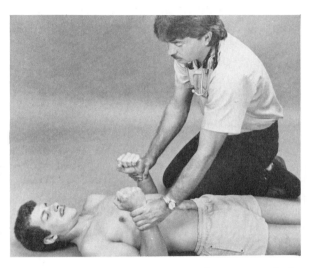

Figure 1.90. Evaluate muscle strength in the upper extremities and compare arms.

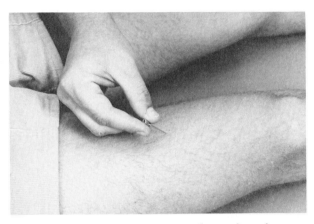

Figure 1.93. Test sensory function in the lower extremity by asking the patient to identify sharp or dull.

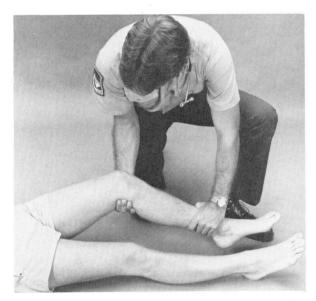

Figure 1.91. Evaluate muscle strength in the lower extremities by comparing both legs.

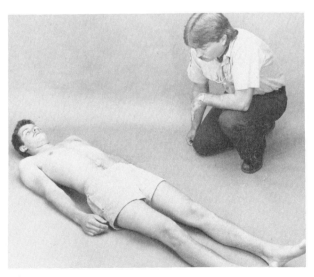

Figure 1.94. Note posture.

unusual posturing. Abnormal findings in posturing are as follows:

1. Decorticate posturing (Figure 1.95). The arms are brought in toward the body (flexed) and the legs are extended. A good way to remember decorticate posturing is that the arms are brought toward the CORE of the body (in deCORticate) as opposed to the arms being extended as in decerebrate posturing. Decorticate

posturing is associated with severe damage to the higher centers of the brain (cortical).

2. Decerebrate posturing (Figure 1.96) is characterized by extension of both the arms and legs, and it has a worse prognosis than decorticate posturing. Decerebrate posturing is associated generally with damage to areas above the brainstem. Generally, all that remains are vegetative functions (respirations, etc.).

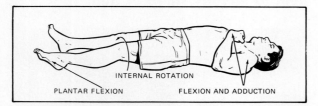

Figure 1.95. Decorticate posturing.

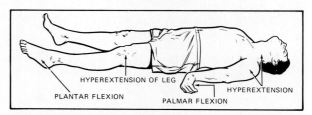

Figure 1.96. Decerebrate posturing.

STUDENT NAME _____ **DATE** _____

DIRECTIONS

Evaluate the student by using the criteria presented on this form. Mark PASS for an appropriate action. Mark FAIL for an inappropriate action or missed step. An asterisk (*) indicates an absolute skill. Omission of this step indicates automatic failure.

	STEP	PASS	FAIL
1.	Quick overview of the total patient	[ ]	[ ]
2.	Quickly evaluate mental status*	[ ]	[ ]
3.	Assess the airway*	[ ]	[ ]
4.	Confirm respirations*	[ ]	[ ]
5.	Confirm circulation*	[ ]	[ ]
6.	Determine level of consciousness	[ ]	[ ]
7.	Determine pulse rate and character*	[ ]	[ ]
8.	Determine respiratory rate*	[ ]	[ ]
9.	Determine blood pressure*	[ ]	[ ]
10.	Inspect and palpate the scalp	[ ]	[ ]
11.	Examination of the face	[ ]	[ ]
12.	Examination of the pupils*	[ ]	[ ]
13.	Inspection of the nose	[ ]	[ ]
14.	Examination of the ears	[ ]	[ ]
15.	Examination of the mouth*	[ ]	[ ]
16.	Examination of the trachea*	[ ]	[ ]
17.	Examination of the carotid pulses	[ ]	[ ]
18.	Examination of the cervical spine*	[ ]	[ ]
19.	Inspection of the chest	[ ]	[ ]
20.	Palpation of the chest*	[ ]	[ ]
21.	Palpate the thoracic spine	[ ]	[ ]
22.	Auscultation of the chest*	[ ]	[ ]
23.	Inspection of the upper extremities	[ ]	[ ]
24.	Palpation of the upper extremities	[ ]	[ ]
25.	Inspection of the nail beds	[ ]	[ ]
26.	Palpation of the radial pulses	[ ]	[ ]
27.	Capillary refill	[ ]	[ ]
28.	Inspect the abdomen	[ ]	[ ]
29.	Palpate the abdomen*	[ ]	[ ]
30.	Palpate the lumbar spine	[ ]	[ ]
31.	Inspect the lower extremities	[ ]	[ ]
32.	Palpate the pelvis	[ ]	[ ]
33.	Palpate the femoral pulses	[ ]	[ ]
34.	Palpate the thigh	[ ]	[ ]
35.	Palpate the leg	[ ]	[ ]
36.	Palpate the pedal pulses	[ ]	[ ]

37.	Test the Babinski reflexes	[ ] [ ]
38.	Test withdrawal to pain	[ ] [ ]
39.	Test motor function in arms	[ ] [ ]
40.	Test motor function in legs	[ ] [ ]
41.	Verbalizes findings properly*	[ ] [ ]
42.	Complete patient report appropriately*	[ ] [ ]

TOTAL SCORE (2 points for each PASS)   ————————
(59 required for PASS)
NO ABSOLUTES MAY BE FAILED

_____

Evaluator   Date

Special Examinations

Several special examinations may be required in various prehospital settings. These examinations are presented separately as they are not a regular part of the paramedic physical examination.

Cranial Nerves

OVERVIEW   Occasionally the EMT/Intermediate (EMT/I) or EMT/Paramedic (EMT/P) may be called upon to evaluate the cranial nerves. Cranial nerves are those nerves that directly leave the brain and go to various parts of the body. Because the cranial nerves exit the skull at different locations, evaluation of these nerves can often be an indicator of such things as increasing intracranial pressure.

There are 12 pairs of cranial nerves (Figure 1.97). Their function is either motor, sensory, or a combination of both. Some nerves, such as the vagus (CN X), also carry parasympathetic fibers. Table 1.5 illustrates the function of the various cranial nerves.

INDICATIONS   Any patient with evidence of neurological deficit where evaluation of cranial nerves is requested by the base station physician.

PRECAUTIONS   When evaluating cranial nerve function find out if any detected cranial nerve deficit was present prior to the current episode.

REQUIRED EQUIPMENT

- Penlight
- Cranial nerve chart
- Sterile needle

PROCEDURE   Evaluation of cranial nerve II (optic nerve) is made by testing vision with a distant object or a vision chart (Figure 1.98).

Cranial nerves III, IV, and VI (oculomotor, trochlear, and abducens) are usually tested together (Figure 1.99). The patient is asked to direct his eyes in six different positions. These positions are referred to as the Cardinal Positions of Gaze.

Cranial nerve V (trigeminal) is evaluated by testing both sensory and motor function in the face (Figure 1.100). Motor function is evaluated by asking the patient to clinch his jaws while you palpate the muscles of mastication. Sensory function is tested by asking the patient to identify sharp or dull.

Table 1.5   The 12 Cranial Nerves and Their Function.

Nerve	Name	Function
I.	Olfactory	smells (not routinely tested)
II.	Optic	sees
III.	Oculomotor	moves eyes
IV.	Trochlear	moves eyes
V.	Trigeminal	sensory to face motor to muscles of mastication
VI.	Abducens	moves eyes
VII.	Facial	motor to muscles of facial expression
VIII.	Acoustic	hearing
IX.	Glossopharyngeal	taste and gag reflex
X.	Vagus	gag reflex and parasympathetic
XI.	Accessory	motor to muscles of neck
XII.	Hypoglossal	motor to tongue

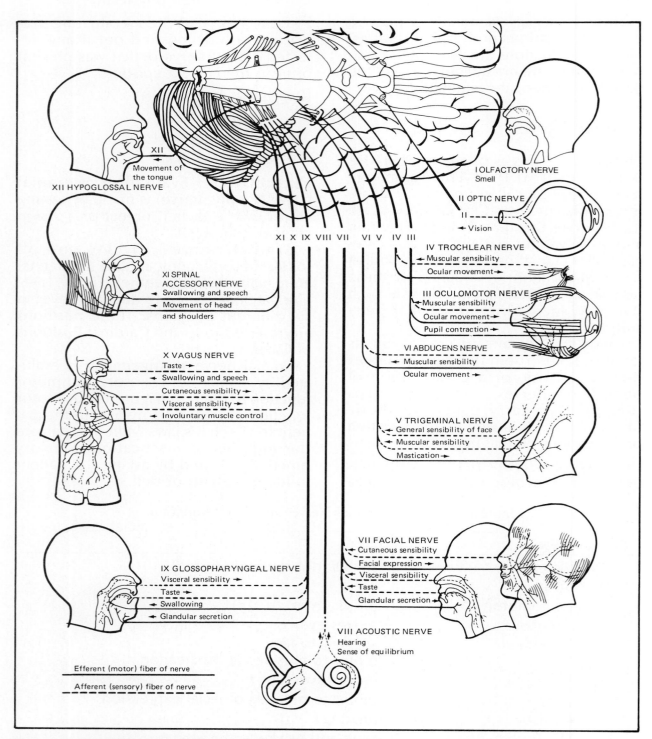

Figure 1.97. Diagram of the 12 pair of cranial nerves.

Cranial nerve VII (facial) is tested by asking the patient to open his eyes against your resistance, to smile, and to show his teeth (Figure 1.101).

Cranial nerve VIII (acoustic) is evaluated by whispering a word some distance from both ears and comparing symmetry (Figure 1.102).

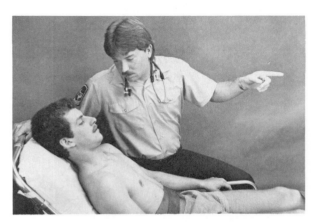

Figure 1.98. Evaluation of cranial nerve II.

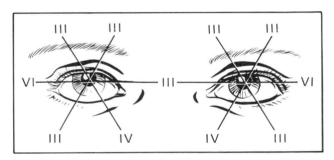

Figure 1.99. Evaluation of cranial nerves III, IV, and VI.

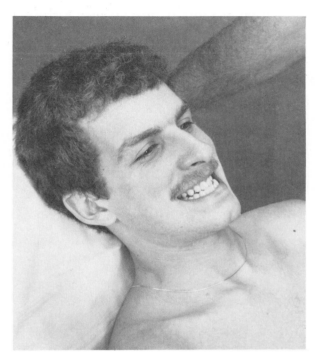

Figure 1.101. Evaluation of cranial nerve VII.

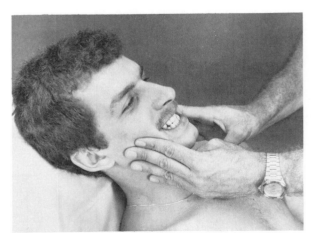

Figure 1.100. Evaluation of cranial nerve V.

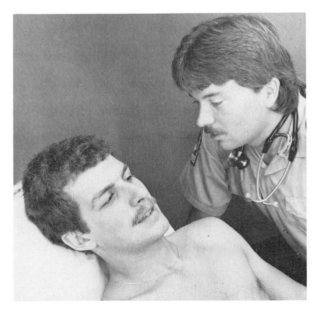

Figure 1.102. Evaluation of cranial nerve VIII.

Cranial nerve IX (glossopharyngeal) (Figure 1.103) is tested by asking the patient to open his mouth and say "ahh." The uvula should be midline, and the palate should elevate symmetrically.

Cranial nerve X (vagus) is evaluated by touching the posteriolateral portion of the pharynx with a tongue blade (Figure 1.104). This should elicit a gag reflex.

Cranial nerve XI (spinal accessory) is tested by asking the patient to shrug his shoulders and turn his head against resistance (Figure 1.105).

Cranial nerve XII (hypoglossal) is evaluated by asking the patient to extend his tongue and move it up, down, left, and right (Figure 1.106).

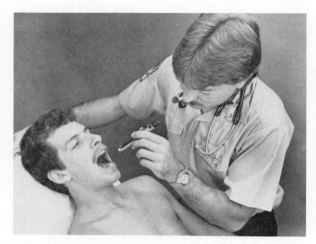

Figure 1.103. Evaluation of cranial nerve IX.

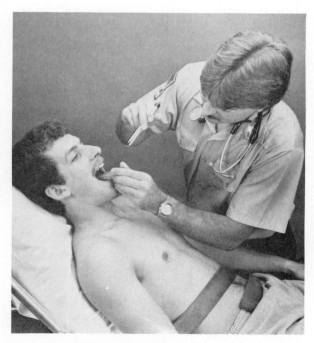

Figure 1.104. Evaluation of cranial nerve X.

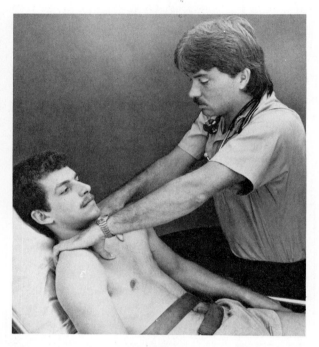

Figure 1.105. Evaluation of cranial nerve XI.

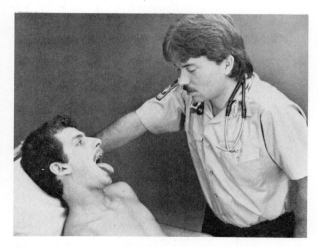

Figure 1.106. Evaluation of cranial nerve XII.

STUDENT NAME —————————————— **DATE** ——————————————

DIRECTIONS

Evaluate the student by using the criteria presented on this form. Mark PASS for an appropriate action. Mark FAIL for an inappropriate action or missed step. ("CN" is cranial nerve.)

STEP	PASS	FAIL
1. Evaluates CN II (optic)	[ ]	[ ]
2. Evaluates CN III, IV, and VI (oculomotor, trochlear, and abducens)	[ ]	[ ]
3. Evaluates CN V (trigeminal)	[ ]	[ ]
4. Evaluates CN VII (facial)	[ ]	[ ]
5. Evaluates CN VIII (acoustic)	[ ]	[ ]
6. Evaluates CN IX (glossopharyngeal)	[ ]	[ ]
7. Evaluates CN X (vagus)	[ ]	[ ]
8. Evaluates CN XI (accessory)	[ ]	[ ]
9. Evaluates CN XII (hypoglossal)	[ ]	[ ]
10. Completes patient report appropriately	[ ]	[ ]

TOTAL SCORE (2 points for each PASS) —————
(14 required for PASS)

—————————————————————— ——————————————
Evaluator   Date

Glassgow Coma Scale

OVERVIEW

The Glassgow Coma Scale has become the accepted standard for the evaluation of patients with suspected neurological injury. It also serves as a systematic method of predicting the long-term prognosis of the patient. The lower the scale, the poorer the long-term prognosis. The Glassgow Coma Scale monitors three parameters: eye opening, best motor response, and verbal response. Each category is graded, and a score is given. The most important use of the Glassgow Coma Scale is to determine whether a patient's neurological status is changing. A worsening of the patient's state is noted when the Glassgow Coma Scale score becomes lower. The method of determining the Glassgow Coma Scale score is detailed in Table 1.6.

INDICATIONS

Any patient with suspected neurological insult or with impaired mental status.

PRECAUTIONS

It is important to note the exact time at which the examination was completed.

REQUIRED EQUIPMENT

None.

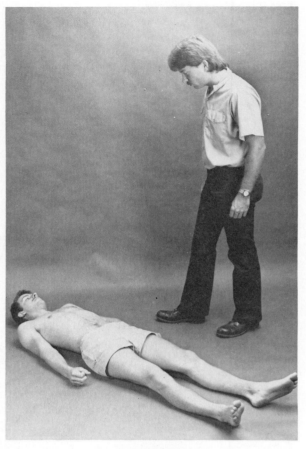

Figure 1.107. Eye opening spontaneous (4 points).

PROCEDURE   First, evaluate eye opening. (Figure 1.107–1.110).

Table 1.6.   The Scoring Method for the Glassgow Coma Scale.

Eye Opening Response	Best Motor Response	Verbal Response
4 = Spontaneous	6 = Obeys	5 = Oriented
3 = To Speech	5 = Localizes	4 = Confused
2 = To Pain	4 = Withdraws	3 = Inappropriate
1 = No Response	3 = Flexion	2 = Sounds
	2 = Extension	1 = No response
	1 = No Response	

Best Possible Score = 15
Worst Possible Score = 3

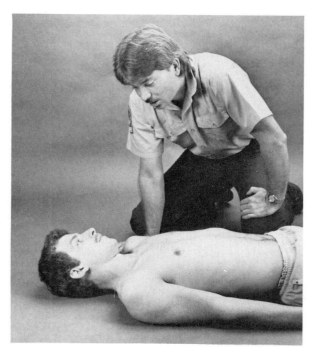

Figure 1.108. Eye opening to speech (3 points).

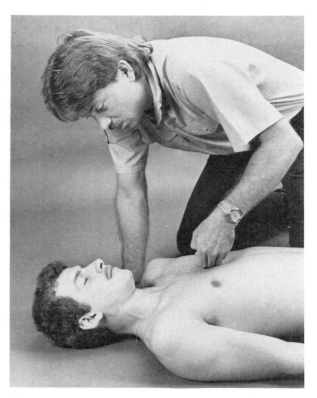

Figure 1.110. No response (1 point).

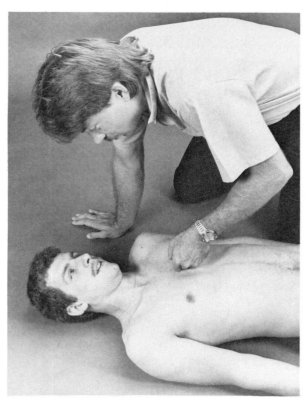

Figure 1.109. Eye opening to pain (2 points).

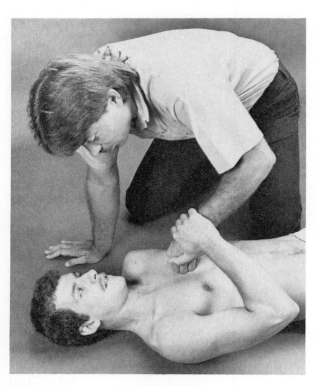

Figure 1.112. Localizes to pain (5 points).

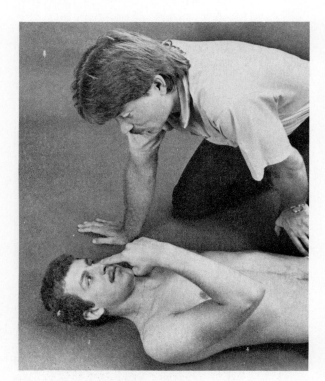

Figure 1.111. Obeys commands (6 points).

Second, evaluate best motor response (Figures 1.111–1.116).

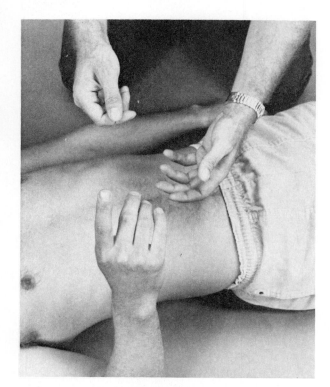

Figure 1.113. Withdraws to pain (4 points).

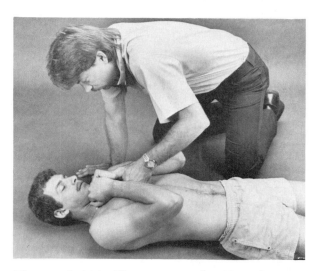

Figure 1.114. Flexes to pain (3 points).

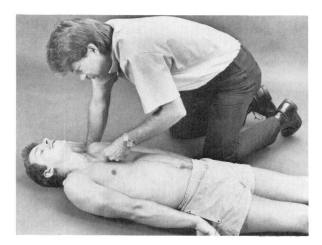

Figure 1.115. Extends to pain (2 points).

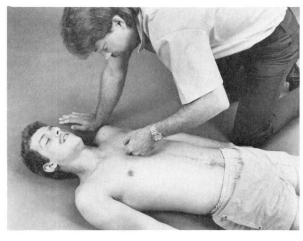

Figure 1.116. No response (1 point).

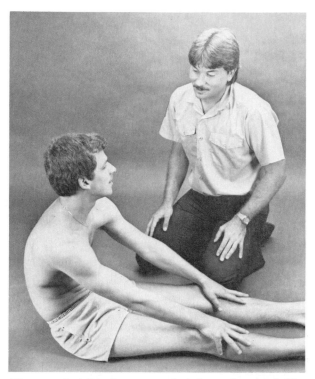

Figure 1.117. Appropriately oriented (5 points).

Last, evaluate verbal response (Figures 1.117–1.121).

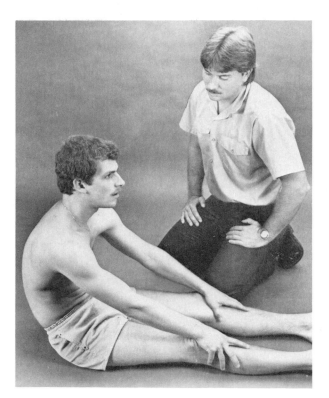

Figure 1.118. Confused conversation (4 points).

47

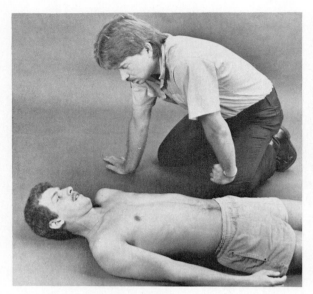

Figure 1.119. Inappropriate words (3 points).

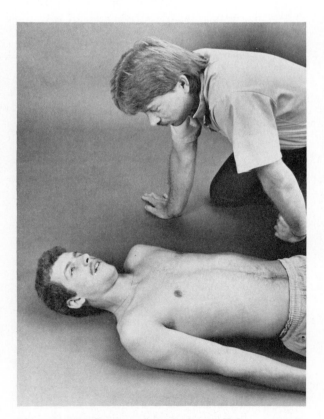

Figure 1.120. Incomprehensible sounds (2 points).

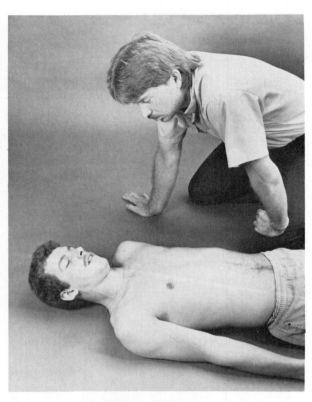

Figure 1.121. No response (1 point).

Assessment

After an adequate amount of both subjective and objective data have been gathered from both the interview and the physical examination, a general assessment of the patient's condition or problem can be made. The term assessment is used in prehospital care as opposed to the term diagnosis because the term diagnosis is used to describe the definitive assessment made by a physician.

Often the patient's problem will be clearly elucidated by the interview and physical examination. However, many cases will occur where the problem is not as evident. Be sure to consider all of the information gained from the interview and physical examination when making an assessment. It is easy to try and jump to conclusions. Case discussion 1 indicates that things are not always as they appear.

Case Discussion 1

Your unit is dispatched to a scene where a patient is complaining of chest pain. The patient, a 52-year-old, white male, states that the pain began while he was watching Monday Night Football. He describes the pain as being substernal with some pain radiating into his left arm. He suffered a myocardial infarction approximately five years ago and is currently taking nitroglycerin and an antihypertensive medication. He took two nitroglycerin tablets approximately 10 minutes before your arrival, and they failed to alleviate his pain. He is overweight and smokes one to two packs of cigarettes a day.

Physical examination reveals a pulse of 100, regular respirations of 22, and a blood pressure of 168/94. ECG reveals no dysrhythmia. The patient is nauseated but not diaphoretic. The chest pain is dull and becomes worse when you press on his chest. The lungs sound clear with the exception of a slight pleural friction rub in the left anterior field.

What is Your Assessment?

Findings at the Emergency Department

The patient was diagnosed as having pleurisy and was discharged from the emergency department approximately two hours after arrival. He was given a prescription for a mild analgesic and an antibiotic.

It is easy to quickly conclude that the patient in Case Discussion 1 was suffering an acute myocardial infarction. However, certain findings such as the friction rub, the apparently normal ECG, and the chest pain worsened by pressure on the chest highly suggest pleuritic chest pain. The point of this discussion is to emphasize that an adequate interview and physical examination are essential to making an appropriate assessment.

When in doubt about what the patient's problem may be, simply give a broad assessment. In Case Discussion 1 the assessment of "Chest Pain rule out (r/o) MI" would be appropriate.

There will be many instances, especially in trauma cases, where more than one problem may be listed in your assessment. These should be listed in the order of severity. Remember that the primary problem may not be the patient's chief complaint. For example, a patient involved in a motor vehicle accident may be bleeding internally. This is the primary problem. However, the primary complaint may be concern with a severely angulated tibia-fibula fracture. Both the chief complaint and the primary problem should be noted.

Plan

The plan is simply the treatment plan devised by yourself and the base-station physician. In cases where only basic life support is indicated, you may not discuss the case with the base-station physician. When formulating a treatment plan you should always list your proposed treatments in the correct order. The following plan would be appropriate for a patient suffering a fractured femur.

1. Administer oxygen at 6 L/min via mask.
2. Maintain body heat.
3. Apply traction splint.
4. Start an IV infusion of lactated Ringer's at 100 mL/hour.
5. Prepare to apply anti-shock trousers.
6. Transport to hospital with orthopedic services.

Initially your plan may be mental. However, for legal reasons and for patient safety, you should write your entire treatment plan on the patient report (Figure 1.122, page 51).

Remember, what was not written on the patient report was not done in a court of law.

Summary

The importance of skilled, accurate, and appropriate patient assessment cannot be overemphasized. The approach to the emergency patient, regardless of the suspected injury or illness, should include a thorough interview and physical examination and an appropriate assessment and treatment plan. This assessment should be presented in the SOAP format, first by gathering SUBJECTIVE DATA, then OBJECTIVE DATA, from which you make an adequate ASSESSMENT which is then followed by an appropriate PLAN.

DALLAS FIRE DEPARTMENT
EMERGENCY MEDICAL SERVICES

PATIENT FORM

FALSE OR
NO TRANSPORT 1 2 3 4 5 6

☑ Dry ☐ Rain ☐ Snow ☐ Ice ☐ Fog
WEATHER CONDITIONS

86-201
INCIDENT NUMBER

1 OF *1*
PATIENTS

Police # ☑ On Scene ☐ Requested   Date *2/15/86*   Time *1530*   Charge _____

Doctor's Name _____   ☐ On Scene ☐ Requested

Location *1601 S. HARWOOD*   Hospital *PARKLAND*

Patient Name *JASON SMITH*   Birthdate *2/21/42*   M ☑ F __ Race *W* Wt *215*
Patient # Assigned at Hosp. If Known *47326-41*

Street *5601 ALLISON*   City & State *DALLAS, TX*   Zip *75021*

Responsible Adult *SAM*   Relationship _____   Phone _____

Drivers License # *0743262 -TX*   Medicare # _____   Medicaid # _____

Employer *City of Dallas*   Soc. Sec. # _____

Paramedic *JOHNSON*   No. *431*   MICU # *704*   Shift *C*

Paramedic/Driver *DeLOACH*   No. *1602*   Responded From *STATION 4*

Vital Signs: B P *110 / 60*   Pulse *84*   Resp. *22*   Allergies *NKA*

Side label: WHITE — Hospital, YELLOW — Tax, PINK — File, GOLD — Paramedic

SEVERITY	TYPE OF INJURY OR ILLNESS		DRUGS	AID PROVIDED BY PARAMEDIC/EMT
Consciousness	1 ☐ Agg. Assault	26 ☐ Medical Emer.	A ☐ Sodium Bicarb	A ☐ EKG
(Con) Semi Unc	2 ☑ Alcohol	27 ☐ Muscle/Skeletal	B ☐ Lidocaine 1%	B ☐ Telemetry
	3 ☐ Asthma	28 ☐ Overdose	C ☐ Lidocaine 4%	C ☑ IV
Bleeding	4 ☑ Auto Accident	29 ☐ Poisoning	D ☐ Atropine	D ☐ Drugs
Non Min (Mod) Sev	5 ☐ Bite/Sting	30 ☐ Psychiatric	E ☐ Isuprel	E ☐ Defib-Suc.
	6 ☐ Burn	31 ☐ Shock	F ☐ Levophed	F ☐ Defib-Unsuc.
Pain	7 ☐ Convulsions	32 ☐ Sickle Cell	G ☐ Epinephrine	G ☐ Esoph-Airway
Non (Min) Mod Sev	8 ☑ Cuts/Bruises	33 ☐ Stabbing	H ☐ Calcium Chl.	H ☐ Intubated
	9 ☐ Diabetic	34 ☐ Stroke	I ☐ Benadryl	I ☑ Oxygen
☐ DOS ☐ DOA	10 ☐ Drowning	35 ☐ Suffocation	J ☐ Valium	J ☐ CPR-Suc.
	11 ☐ Drug Reaction	36 ☐ Suicide	K ☐ Dextrose 50%	K ☐ CPR-Unsuc.
LOCATION OF INJURY-ILLNESS	12 ☐ Dyspnea	37 ☐ T.B.	L ☐ Nitronox	L ☐ Cont. Bleed
☑ Head	13 ☐ Electrocution	38 ☐ VD	M ☐ Narcan	M ☑ Bandaging
☐ Face	14 ☐ Emer. Trans.	39 ☐ None	N ☐ Alcaine	N ☑ Splinting
☐ Eye L/R	15 ☐ Emphysema	40 ☐ Other (Specify)	O ☐ Ipecac	O ☐ Spine Board
☐ Neck	16 ☐ Fainted		P ☐ Burn Spray	P ☐ Anti-Shock
☐ Back	17 ☐ Female Comp.		Q ☐ Epine. 1:1000	Q ☐ OB-Live Br.
☑ Chest	18 ☐ Flu	**RESPONSE CODE TO HOSPITAL**	R ☐ Lasix	R ☐ OB-Still Br.
☐ Abdomen	19 ☑ Fracture		S ☐ Bretylol	S ☐ Rotating TK
☐ Pelvic Region	20 ☐ GI Complaint	☑ 1		T ☐ Trans. Only
☑ Upper Extremity (L)R	21 ☐ Gunshot	☐ 3		U ☐ None
☐ Lower Extremity L/R	22 ☐ Heart			V ☐ Other
☐ Respiratory	23 ☐ Hypervent.		**IV**	W ☐ CPR Citizen
☐ Cardiovascular	24 ☐ Hypoglycemia		1 ☑ Ringers Lac.	X ☐ CPR Thumper
☐ Other	25 ☐ Maternity		2 ☐ D5W	Y ☐ MAST Trousers
				Z ☐ Dextrostix

Chief Complaint *Multiple cuts & fractures 2° TO MVA*   Aid Provided By

Remarks *Pt. involved in 2 car MVA. Driver of car struck on ©. Trapped for 15 minutes.*   Fire Co. # *3*

Other _____

If Interhospital Transfer, ER Doctor authorizing move: _____

I was offered aid by the City of Dallas Emergency Medical Service. I chose not to accept Emergency Treatment and/or Transportation

Signature _____   Witness _____

Doctor or R.N. signature below does not approve or disapprove above information

DFD Form 200 Revised SEP 80   FRD-00981   Dr. or R.N. _____
SIGNATURE ACCEPTING PATIENT

Figure 1.122. Completed patient report showing proper reporting of a thorough advanced patient assessment with an appropriate plan.

Chapter Objectives

Upon completion of this chapter, the student should be able to:

1. List the indications, contraindications, precautions, and common complications of the following procedures:

   a. Placement of an esophageal obturator airway

   b. Placement of an esophageal obturator airway with gastric tube

   c. Adult endotracheal intubation

   d. Pediatric endotracheal intubation

   e. Endotracheal intubation with esophageal obturator airway (EOA) in place

   f. Nasotracheal intubation

   g. Blind nasotracheal intubation

   h. Tracheal suctioning

   i. Airway clearance with McGill forceps

   j. Cricothyrotomy

2. Be able to perform the following procedures according to the criteria presented:

   a. Placement of an esophageal obturator airway

   b. Placement of an esophageal obturator airway gastric tube

   c. Adult endotracheal intubation

   d. Pediatric endotracheal intubation

   e. Endotracheal intubation with EOA in place

   f. Nasotracheal intubation

   g. Blind nasotracheal intubation

   h. Tracheal suctioning

   i. Airway clearance with McGill forceps

   j. Cricothyrotomy

2

Airway Management Skills

Placement of the Esophageal Obturator Airway

Overview

The esophageal obturator airway (EOA) is an adjunctive airway device designed to be inserted without visualization of the airway (Figure 2.1). The tube, which has a closed end, is placed in the esophagus. When in place, the cuff is inflated, and the esophagus is effectively obstructed. When the patient is ventilated air is forced into the trachea.

Indications

Deep coma, respiratory arrest, or cardiopulmonary arrest as noted by apnea or lack of gag reflex.

Contraindications

1. Patients under 16 years of age.
2. Patients with a history of esophageal disease.
3. Patients who have ingested a strong base, a strong acid, or a petroleum distillate.

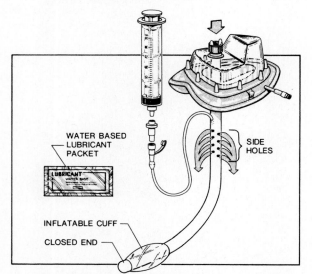

Figure 2.1. Esophageal obturator airway (EOA).

WATER BASED
LUBRICANT
PACKET

LUBRICANT
WATER BASE

SIDE
HOLES

INFLATABLE CUFF

CLOSED END

4. Any patient with a gag reflex.
5. Patients less than 5 feet or greater than 7 feet tall.
6. Severe oral or nasal bleeding.

Precautions

The EOA should never be left in place for more than 2 hours. If a patient requires prolonged ventilation then endotracheal intubation should be performed.

An adequate seal must be maintained at all times with the mask. Also, the seal on the mask should be checked frequently (usually with the daily vehicle and equipment check) and reinflated if necessary.

Vomiting commonly accompanies the removal of the EOA. Because of this, endotracheal intubation should precede EOA extubation when possible. In either case, vomiting should be anticipated, and the patient should be placed on his or her side prior to removal. **SUCTION MUST BE AVAILABLE.**

Complications

1. Esophageal tears
2. Ruptured esophageal varices
3. Accidental intubation of trachea

Required Equipment

● Esophageal obturator airway
● 35-mL Syringe
● Water-soluble lubricant
● Suction

Procedure

Prepare Equipment

Inflate the mask (Figure 2.2).
Test the mask seal (Figure 2.3).
Inflate the cuff (Figure 2.4)
Test the cuff (Figure 2.5).
Deflate the cuff (Figure 2.6).

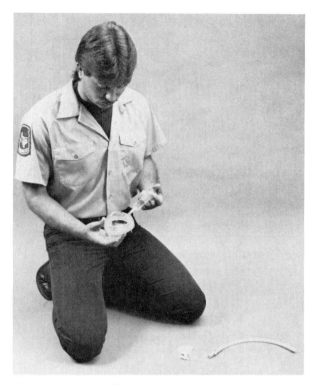

Figure 2.2. Inflate the mask.

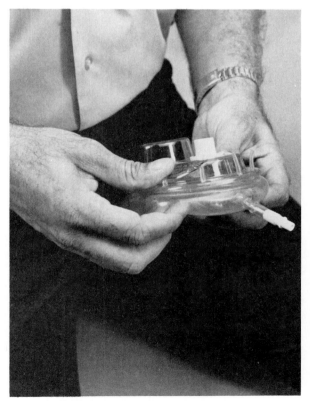

Figure 2.3. Test the mask seal.

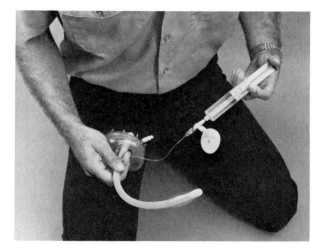

Figure 2.4. Inflate the cuff.

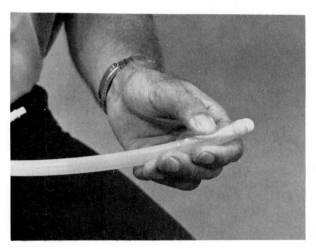

Figure 2.5. Test the cuff.

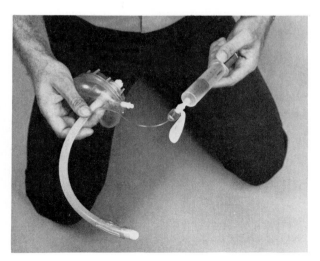

Figure 2.6. Deflate the cuff.

Insertion of the Airway

Apply water-soluble lubricant to the tip and cuff (Figure 2.7).

Hyperventilate the patient in anticipation of EOA insertion (Figure 2.8).

Position the patient with head slightly flexed unless a C-spine injury has not been ruled out (Figure 2.9).

Insert the airway (Figures 2.10–2.12).

Check placement by auscultating the chest and watching for it to rise (Figure 2.13).

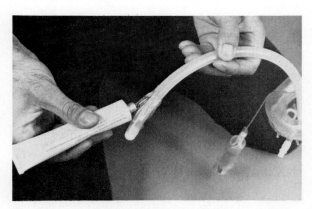

Figure 2.7. Apply lubricant to tip and cuff.

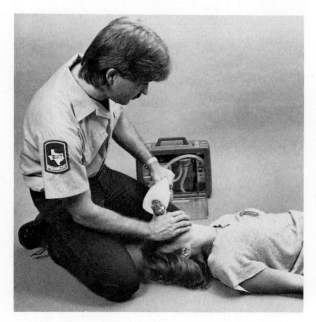

Figure 2.8. Patient hyperventilation.

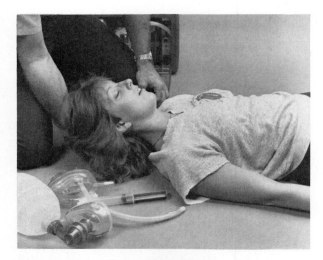

Figure 2.9. Patient position.

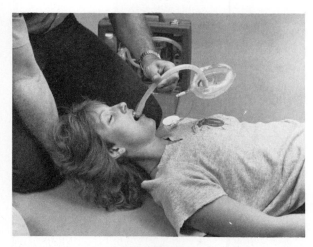

Figure 2.10. Begin airway insertion.

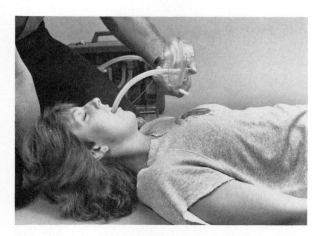

Figure 2.11. Airway in the middle of insertion.

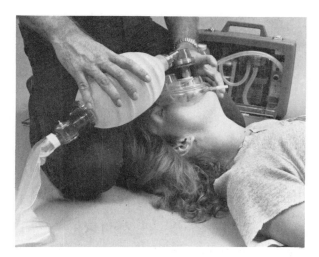

Figure 2.12. Airway in position.

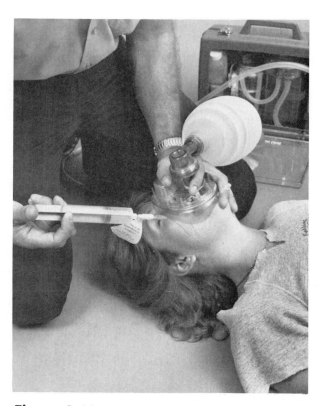

Figure 2.14.

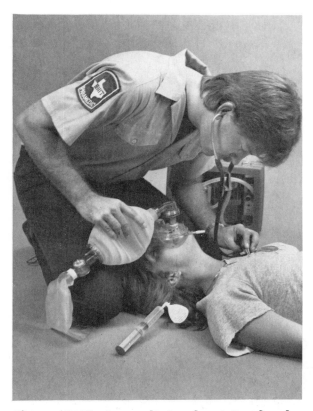

Figure 2.13. Auscultate chest to check placement.

Inflate the cuff with the quantity of air directed by the manufacturer (Figure 2.14).

Auscultate the chest and abdomen (Figure 2.15).

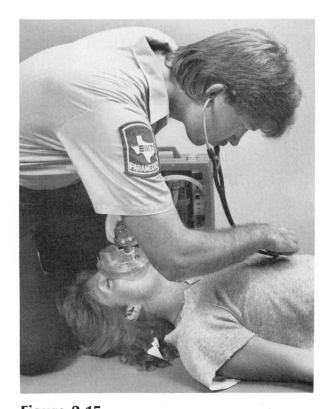

Figure 2.15.

Removal of EOA

Turn the patient on his side if C-spine injury is not suspected (Figure 2.16).

Deflate the cuff (Figure 2.17).

Remove mask and insert suction catheter (Figure 2.18).

Withdraw airway while maintaining suction (Figure 2.19).

Examine the mouth for any foreign material before returning patient to supine position (Figure 2.20).

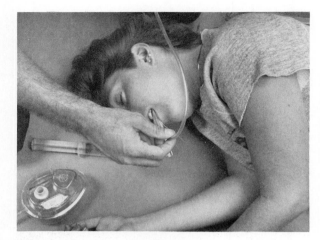

Figure 2.18.

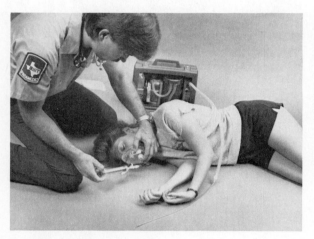

Figure 2.16.

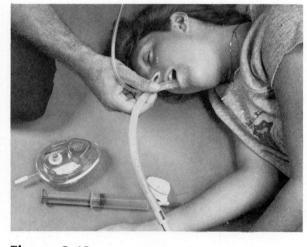

Figure 2.19.

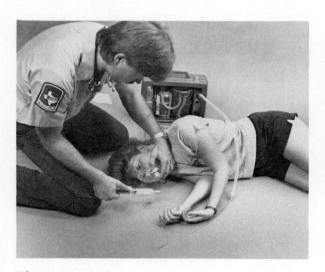

Figure 2.17.

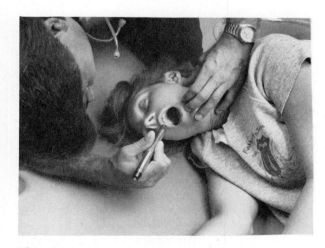

Figure 2.20.

STUDENT NAME ————————————————— **DATE** —————————

DIRECTIONS

Evaluate the student by using the criteria presented on this form. Mark PASS for an appropriate action. Mark FAIL for an inappropriate action or missed step. An asterisk (*) indicates an absolute step. Omission of this step indicates automatic failure.

STEP	PASS	FAIL
1. Tests mask seal*	[ ]	[ ]
2. Inflates and tests cuff*	[ ]	[ ]
3. Deflates cuff	[ ]	[ ]
4. Applies lubricant to tip of EOA	[ ]	[ ]
5. Hyperventilates patient*	[ ]	[ ]
6. Positions patient's head properly*	[ ]	[ ]
7. Inserts EOA properly	[ ]	[ ]
8. Checks placement*	[ ]	[ ]
9. Inflates cuff with 35 mL of air	[ ]	[ ]
10 Ventilates patient*	[ ]	[ ]
11 Auscultates chest and abdomen*	[ ]	[ ]
Removal of EOA		
12. Determines level of consciousness	[ ]	[ ]
13. Prepares equipment for removal	[ ]	[ ]
14. Turns patient on side*	[ ]	[ ]
15. Deflates cuff*	[ ]	[ ]
16. Removes mask (inserts ET if required)	[ ]	[ ]
17. Inserts suction catheter into mouth	[ ]	[ ]
18. Withdraws airway while maintaining suction	[ ]	[ ]
19. Examines mouth for foreign material	[ ]	[ ]
20. Completes written report properly	[ ]	[ ]

TOTAL SCORE (2 points for each pass) —————
(28 required for PASS)
NO ABSOLUTES MAY BE FAILED

——————————————————   ——————————————————
Evaluator   Date

Placement of the Esophageal Obturator Airway with Gastric Tube

Overview

The esophageal obturator airway with gastric tube (EGTA) (Figure 2.21) is useful in reducing abdominal distension and is useful in reducing the amount of vomiting that accompanies removal of the EOA. The EGTA ventilates through a port in the mask as opposed to the EOA which ventilates through holes in the tube. The port where the bag–valve–mask unit attaches to the EGTA is in a different location than the port on the standard EOA.

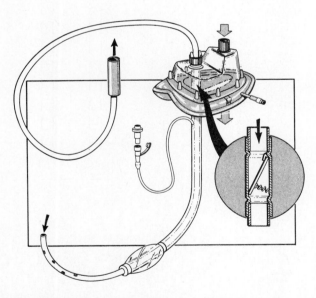

Figure 2.21. Esophageal obturator airway with gastric tube.

Indications

Deep coma, respiratory arrest, or cardiopulmonary arrest as evidenced by apnea or the absence of a gag reflex.

Contraindications

1. Patients under 16 years of age.
2. Patients with a history of esophageal disease.
3. Patients who have ingested a strong base, a strong acid, or a petroleum distillate.
4. Any patient with a gag reflex.
5. Patients less than 5 feet or greater than 7 feet tall.
6. Severe oral or nasal bleeding.

Precautions

The same precautions apply to the EGTA as apply to the standard EOA.

Complications

1. Esophageal tears
2. Ruptured esophageal varices
3. Accidental intubation of the trachea
4. Irritation of the gastric mucosa

Required Equipment

Esophageal obturator airway with gastric tube
Water-soluble lubricant
35-mL Syringe
Suction

Procedure

The procedure for inserting the EGTA tube is the same as the standard EOA. However, the following variations in the skills sequence apply:

- After tube placement is checked by auscultation, insert the gastric tube into the opening (Figure 2.22).
- Insert the gastric tube to the point marked on the tube (Figure 2.23)
- If required, attach the tube to suction device (Figure 2.24).

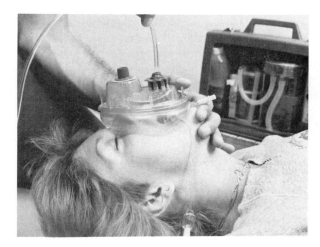

Figure 2.22.

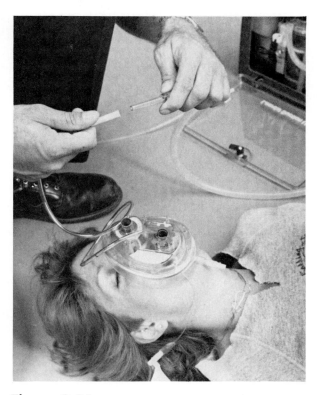

Figure 2.24.

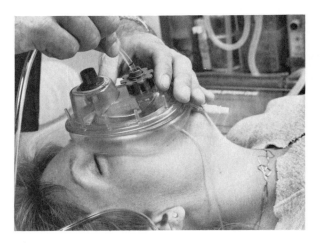

Figure 2.23.

STUDENT NAME _____ **DATE** _____

DIRECTIONS

Evaluate the student by using the criteria presented on this form. Mark PASS for an appropriate action. Mark FAIL for an inappropriate action or missed step. An asterisk (*) indicates an absolute step. Omission of this step indicates automatic failure.

	STEP	PASS	FAIL
1.	Tests mask seal*	[ ]	[ ]
2.	Inflates and tests cuff*	[ ]	[ ]
3.	Deflates cuff	[ ]	[ ]
4.	Applies lubricant to tip of EGTA	[ ]	[ ]
5.	Hyperventilates patient*	[ ]	[ ]
6.	Positions patient's head properly*	[ ]	[ ]
7.	Inserts EGTA properly	[ ]	[ ]
8.	Checks placement*	[ ]	[ ]
9.	Inflates cuff with 35 mL of air	[ ]	[ ]
10.	Ventilates patient*	[ ]	[ ]
11.	Auscultates chest and abdomen*	[ ]	[ ]
12.	Inserts gastric tube in airway	[ ]	[ ]
13.	Inserts gastric tube to mark on tube	[ ]	[ ]
14.	Maintains ventilations*	[ ]	[ ]
15.	Completes written report properly	[ ]	[ ]

TOTAL SCORE (2 points for each pass)
(21 required for PASS)   _____
NO ABSOLUTES MAY BE FAILED

_____   _____
                    Evaluator   Date

Adult Endotracheal Intubation

Overview

Endotracheal intubation is the placement of a tube into the trachea. It is the preferred method of airway maintenance in the unconscious patient.

Indications

1. Patients in deep coma, respiratory arrest, or cardiopulmonary arrest.
2. Patients where complete obstruction of the airway appears imminent (for example, respiratory burns).
3. Patients where tracheal suctioning is required to remove material that may be critically blocking the airway.

Contraindications

1. Patients with an intact gag reflex.
2. Patients where irritation of the pharynx might cause laryngeal spasm (for example, croup or epiglottitis)

Precautions

Endotracheal intubation is a skill that requires adequate training first on mannikins, then on cadavers, and finally in the operating room. It is a skill that can rapidly decay without adequate usage or refresher training.

It is important not to take longer than 15 seconds per attempt. If it appears that the attempt will exceed 15 seconds then you should stop and hyperventilate the patient before trying again. A good way to remember this is to hold your own breath while attempting intubation. This acts as a kind of subconscious reminder.

Other techniques of airway management may be indicated if there is a suspected injury to the cervical spine since endotracheal intubation requires extension of the head. In these cases, if a second rescuer is available, have that person maintain the neck in a neutral position while endotracheal intubation is attempted.

If vomiting occurs during endotracheal intubation the reverse peristaltic wave can frequently be suppressed by pressure below the thyroid cartilage on the cricopharyngeus muscle.

The importance of verifying successful endotracheal intubation by auscultation of the chest following the procedure cannot be overemphasized. Accidental intubation of the esophagus, resulting in prolonged hypoxia, is usually always fatal if not quickly remedied.

Complications

1. Accidental intubation of the esophagus.
2. Insertion of the endotracheal tube too far (endobronchial intubation).
3. Oropharyngeal trauma.
4. Fractured teeth or dentures.
5. Spasm of the vocal chords

Required Equipment

- Endotracheal tube
- Lubricant
- Stylet
- 10-mL Syringe
- Laryngoscope blade
- Laryngoscope handle
- McGill forceps
- 1-inch Adhesive tape

The endotracheal tube (Figure 2.25) is a curved tube with a balloon cuff at the distal end and a 15-mm adapter at the proximal end. The balloon cuff holds approximately 5–10 mL of air.

Endotracheal tubes are sized on the basis of diameter of the tube. Normally, an adult male will require a 7.5–8.5-mm

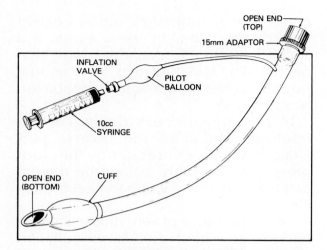

Figure 2.25. Cuffed endotracheal tube.

endotracheal tube. An adult female will normally require a 7.0–8.0-mm tube.

Two types of laryngoscope blades are used in prehospital care. These are the Miller-Abbott or straight blade (Figure 2.26) and the McIntosh or curved blade. The blades attach to a laryngoscope handle which provides the power source for the light.

The straight blade is used to actually lift the epiglottis (Figures 2.27–2.29).

The curved blade (Figure 2.30), on the other hand, fits into the area above the epiglottis referred to as the vallecula (Figure 2.31). Upward pressure on the

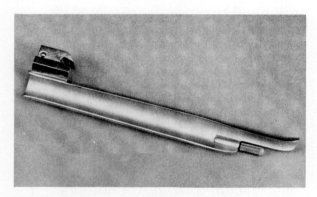

Figure 2.26. Straight laryngoscope blade.

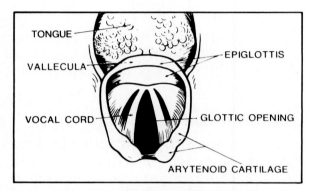

Figure 2.28. Anatomy of the glottic opening.

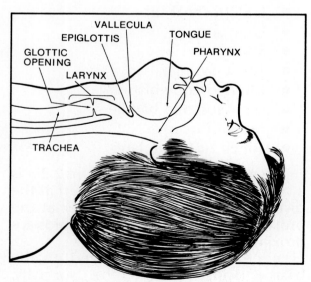

Figure 2.27. Anatomy of the pharynx.

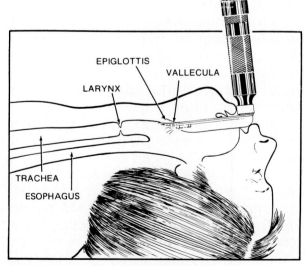

Figure 2.29. Straight laryngoscope blade in place in the laryngopharynx.

vallecula elevates the epiglottis, thus exposing the laryngeal opening.

The laryngoscope blade attaches to the handle by first engaging the blade (Figure 2.32) and then elevating it into position (Figure 2.33).

The stylet is an important part of the endotracheal intubation kit. It is used to hold the endotracheal tube into optimal shape during intubation. The best method is to place the stylet into the endotracheal tube and shape the tube in the shape of a "hockey stick" (Figure 2.34).

A stylet with a ball on the end is preferred. The stylet should not extend past the tip of the tube.

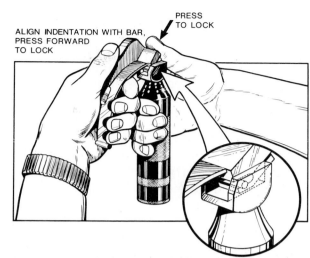

Figure 2.32. Engaging the laryngoscope blade.

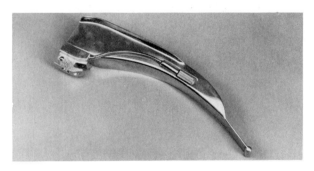

Figure 2.30. Curved laryngoscope blade.

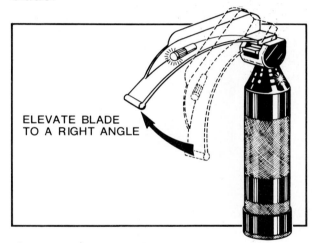

Figure 2.33. Elevating the laryngoscope blade to turn on light source.

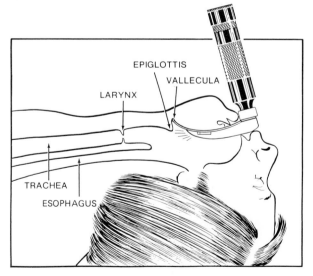

Figure 2.31. Curved laryngoscope blade properly placed in the vallecula.

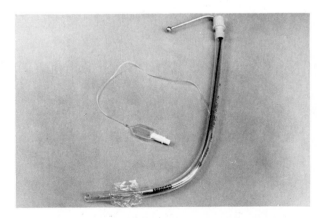

Figure 2.34. Endotracheal tube with a stylet in place and shaped into "hockey stick" configuration.

The McGill forceps are only occasionally used. They are good for removing foreign bodies and for lifting the end of the endotracheal tube in patients with anteriorly displaced laryngeal openings.

Procedure

PREPARE AND CHECK EQUIPMENT

Inflate the cuff on the endotracheal tube (ET) to test (Figure 2.35).

Deflate the cuff (Figure 2.36).

Check laryngoscope light (Figure 2.37).

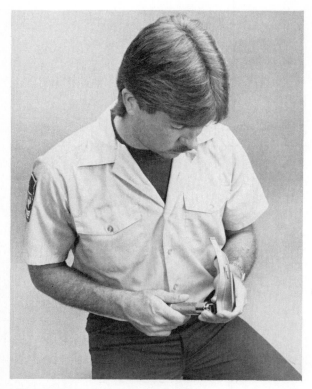

Figure 2.37.

TECHNIQUE

Hyperventilate the patient (Figure 2.38).

Place the patient in the "sniffing position" with the head extended (Figure 2.39).

Hold laryngoscope in the left hand (Figure 2.40).

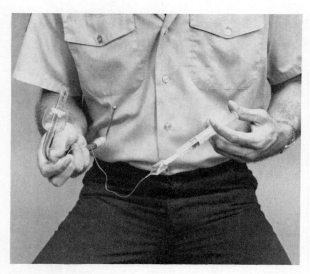

Figure 2.35.

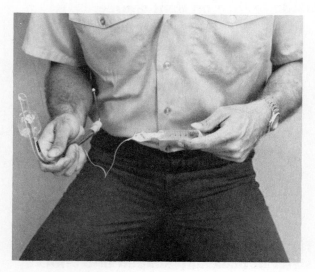

Figure 2.36.

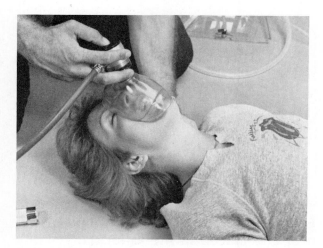

Figure 2.38.

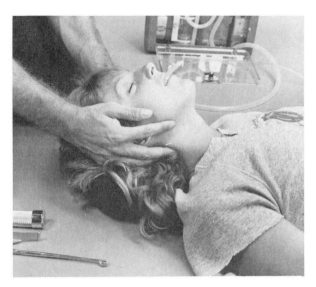

Figure 2.39. The "sniffing position."

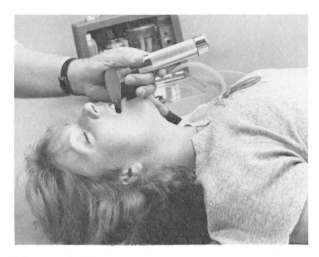

Figure 2.41.

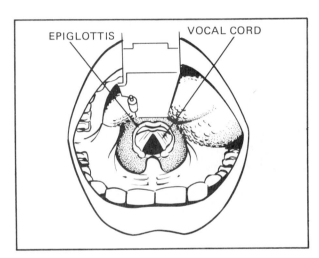

EPIGLOTTIS   VOCAL CORD

Figure 2.42.

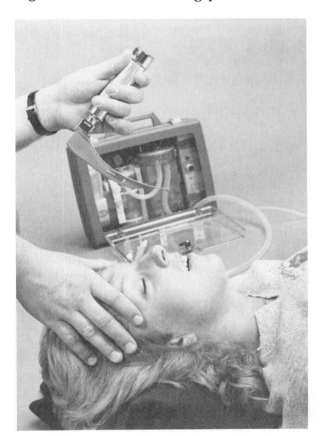

Figure 2.40.

Insert the laryngoscope blade (Figure 2.41).
Visualize the vocal cords (Figure 2.42).
Insert ET tube (Figure 2.43).

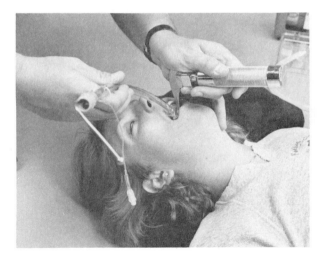

Figure 2.43.

Maintain visualization as tube passes through laryngeal opening (Figure 2.44).

Remove the laryngoscope blade (Figure 2.45).

Ventilate and check tube placement (Figure 2.46).

Inflate the balloon cuff with 5–10 mL of air or until met with resistance (Figure 2.47).

Auscultate both the chest and abdomen (Figure 2.48).

Add an oropharyngeal airway (Figure 2.49).

Tape the tube (Figure 2.50).

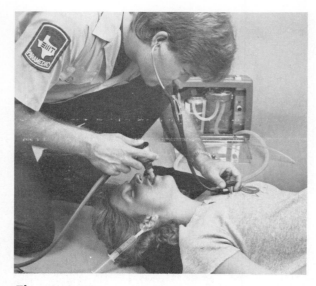

Figure 2.46.

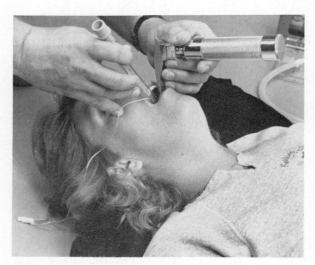

Figure 2.44.

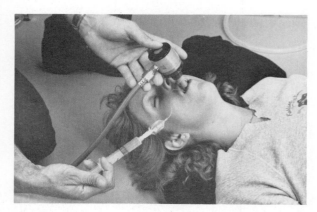

Figure 2.47.

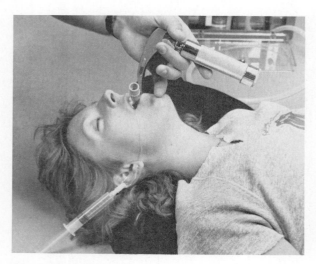

Figure 2.45.

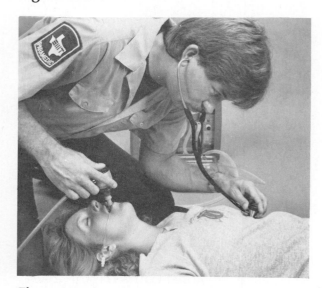

Figure 2.48.

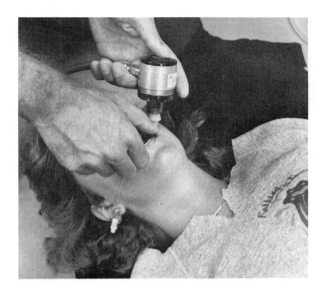

Figure 2.49.

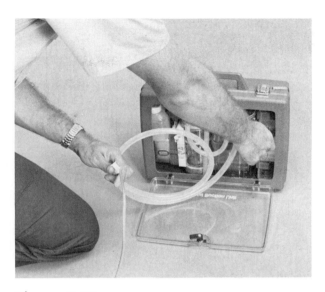

Figure 2.51.

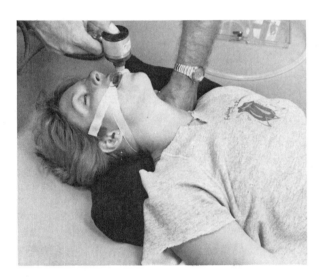

Figure 2.50.

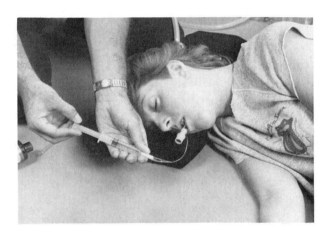

Figure 2.52.

Extubation

An endotracheal tube can be removed when the patient is conscious enough to maintain his own airway. This procedure should be deferred until the patient is in the emergency department and has been evaluated by the emergency physician.

Have suction available (Figure 2.51).
Deflate the cuff (Figure 2.52).
Extubate during inspiration (Figure 2.53).

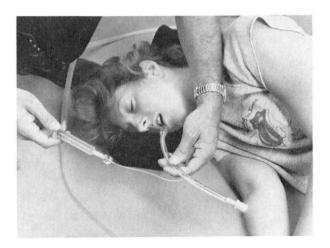

Figure 2.53.

STUDENT NAME _____ **DATE** _____

DIRECTIONS

Evaluate the student by using the criteria presented on this form. Mark PASS for an appropriate action. Mark FAIL for an inappropriate action or missed step. An asterisk (*) indicates an absolute step. Omission of this step indicates automatic failure.

	STEP	PASS	FAIL
1.	Tests cuff*	[ ]	[ ]
2.	Deflates cuff*	[ ]	[ ]
3.	Checks laryngoscope and light*	[ ]	[ ]
4.	Selects appropriate blade	[ ]	[ ]
5.	Hyperventilates patient*	[ ]	[ ]
6.	Places patient in "sniffing position"*	[ ]	[ ]
7.	Holds laryngoscope in left hand*	[ ]	[ ]
8.	Inserts laryngoscope properly*	[ ]	[ ]
9.	Does not use teeth as a fulcrum*	[ ]	[ ]
10.	Visualizes cords*	[ ]	[ ]
11.	Inserts appropriate size ET tube	[ ]	[ ]
12.	Maintains visualization as tube is passed	[ ]	[ ]
13.	Removes laryngoscope blade	[ ]	[ ]
14.	Checks tube placement*	[ ]	[ ]
15.	Inflates cuff with an 5–10 mL of air	[ ]	[ ]
16.	Auscultates chest and abdomen*	[ ]	[ ]
17.	Adds oropharyngeal airway	[ ]	[ ]
18.	Tapes tube	[ ]	[ ]
19.	Completes in 15 seconds*	[ ]	[ ]
	EXTUBATION		
20.	Tests level of consciousness	[ ]	[ ]
21.	Turns patient's head to side	[ ]	[ ]
22.	Deflates cuff	[ ]	[ ]
23.	Removes ET tube	[ ]	[ ]
24.	Extubates during expiration	[ ]	[ ]
25.	Reassesses airway	[ ]	[ ]

TOTAL SCORE (2 points for each PASS)   _____
(35 required for PASS)
NO ABSOLUTES MAY BE FAILED

_____   _____
Evaluator   Date

Pediatric Endotracheal Intubation

Overview

Pediatric endotracheal intubation is essentially the same procedure as adult endotracheal intubation. Generally the straight laryngoscope blade is preferred over the curved. If a pediatric size blade (that is a #1 or a #2) is not available, then an adult straight blade (#3 or #4) may be used. However, caution should be taken not to insert the blade too far which could conceivably damage the vocal cords. Uncuffed endotracheal tubes are preferred in children because of the narrow diameter of the trachea. Table 2-1 illustrates common endotracheal tube sizes for children.

Table 2-1. Common Endotracheal Tube Sizes for Children

Approximate Age	Internal Diameter (mm)
Small newborn (< 1kg)	2.5
Newborn–6 months	3.0–3.5
6 months–1 year	3.5–4.0
1–3 years	4.0–5.0
3–5 years	5.0–5.5
5–7 years	5.5–6.0
8–10 years	6.0–6.5
11–12 years	6.5–7.0
12–17 years	7.0–8.5

A good rule of thumb for estimating endotracheal tube sizes in children up to 7 years is to use a tube of approximately the same outside diameter as the little finger of the child.

Indications

Same as adult endotracheal intubation.

Contraindications

Same as adult endotracheal intubation.

Precautions

Same as adult endotracheal intubation.

Complications

Same as adult endotracheal intubation.

Required Equipment

- Uncuffed endotracheal tube
- Small stylet
- Lubricant
- 1-inch Adhesive tape
- Laryngoscope handle
- #1 or #2 Straight blade

Procedure

Prepare equipment (Figure 2.54).

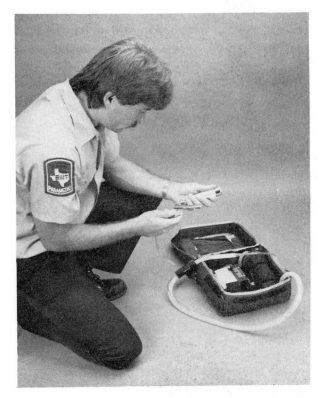

Figure 2.54.

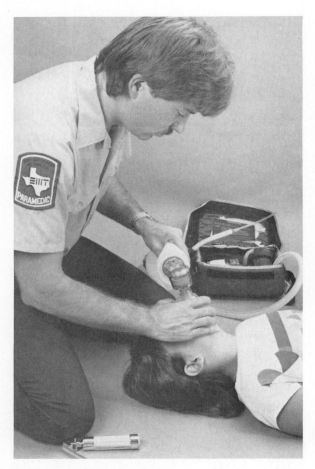

Figure 2.55.

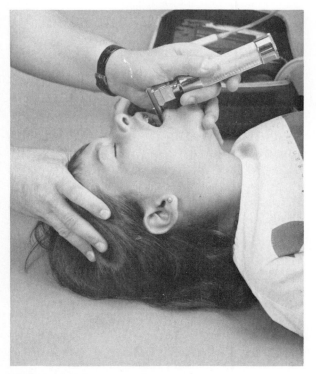

Figure 2.56.

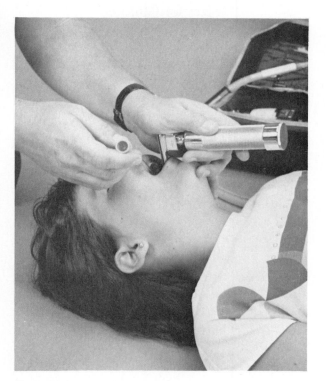

Figure 2.57.

Hyperventilate the child (Figure 2.55).

Insert the laryngoscope blade (Figure 2.56).

Insert the endotracheal tube (Figure 2.57).

Ventilate and check tube placement (Figure 2.58).

Ventilate with a bag–valve–mask unit (Figure 2.59).

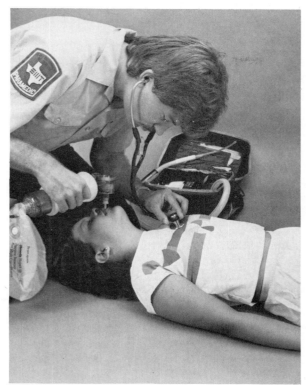

Figure 2.58.

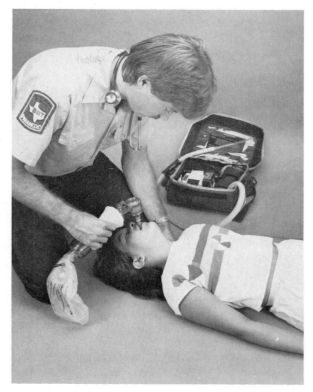

Figure 2.59.

STUDENT NAME _____ **DATE** _____

DIRECTIONS

Evaluate the student by using the criteria presented on this form. Mark PASS for an appropriate action. Mark FAIL for an inappropriate action or missed step. An asterisk (*) indicates an absolute step. Omission of this step indicates automatic failure.

	STEP	PASS	FAIL
1.	Checks laryngoscope and light*	[ ]	[ ]
2.	Selects appropriate blade	[ ]	[ ]
3.	Hyperventilates child*	[ ]	[ ]
4.	Inserts laryngoscope blade properly	[ ]	[ ]
5.	Does not use teeth as fulcrum*	[ ]	[ ]
6.	Inserts endotracheal tube while maintaining visualization of vocal cords.	[ ]	[ ]
7.	Checks tube placement*	[ ]	[ ]
8.	Ventilates patient*	[ ]	[ ]
9.	Auscultates chest*	[ ]	[ ]
10.	Secures tube	[ ]	[ ]
11.	Takes no longer than 15 seconds or attempts to reventilate*	[ ]	[ ]

TOTAL SCORE (2 points for each PASS)   _____
(15 required for PASS)
NO ABSOLUTES MAY BE FAILED

_____   _____
Evaluator   Date

Endotracheal Intubation with EOA in Place

Overview

The esophageal obturator airway (EOA) is not designed for long-term airway maintenance. Patients who require prolonged airway management should have an endotracheal tube placed. The endotracheal tube is best inserted while the EOA is still in place. This procedure has several advantages. First, the EOA is often a superior way of managing the patient's airway until endotracheal intubation can be performed. Second, the EOA usually prevents vomiting during endotracheal intubation making the procedure much easier for the operator and safer for the patient. Third, with the EOA placed properly in the esophagus, the laryngeal opening is often much easier to identify. Finally, because removal of the EOA is often accompanied by vomiting, placement of the endotracheal tube protects the airway and prevents possible aspiration.

Indications

1. Deep coma, respiratory arrest, or cardiopulmonary arrest where prolonged ventilation is indicated.
2. Cases where the EOA fails to function properly or the contour of the patient's face prohibits an adequate mask seal.
3. Cases where abdominal distension is not prevented by the EOA, and gastric suctioning is required.

Contraindications

1. Patients where irritation of the pharynx might induce laryngeal spasm (for example, croup or epiglottitis).
2. Patients with substantial oral trauma.

Precautions

It is important to take no longer than 15–20 seconds to perform this procedure. If it appears that the attempt will take longer than 15 seconds, then the mask should be replaced on the EOA, and the patient should be ventilated.

Assure that the endotracheal tube is properly in place and the cuff is sufficiently inflated before removing the EOA as vomitus might pass the cuff and enter the trachea.

Complications

1. Accidental intubation of the esophagus.
2. Insertion of the endotracheal tube too far (endobronchial intubation).
3. Oropharyngeal trauma.
4. Fractured teeth or dentures.
5. Spasm of the vocal cords.

Required Equipment

*   Endotracheal tube
*   Lubricant
*   Stylet
*   10-mL Syringe
*   Laryngoscope blade
*   Laryngoscope handle
*   McGill forceps
*   1-inch Adhesive tape

Procedure

PREPARE AND CHECK EQUIPMENT
Test the cuff on the endotracheal tube (Figure 2.60).
Prepare equipment (Figure 2.61).

INSERTION OF AN EOA
Hyperventilate the patient (Figure 2.62).
Remove EOA mask (Figure 2.63).
Move EOA tube, inflation tube, and balloon to the left side of patient's mouth (Figure 2.64).

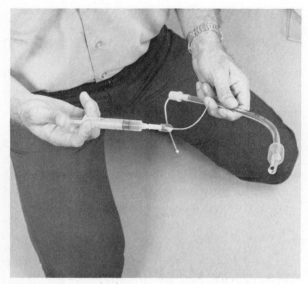

Figure 2.60.

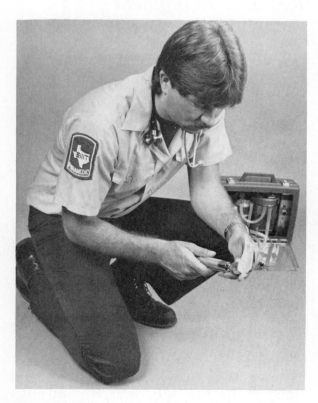

Figure 2.61.

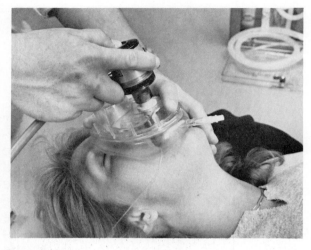

Figure 2.62.

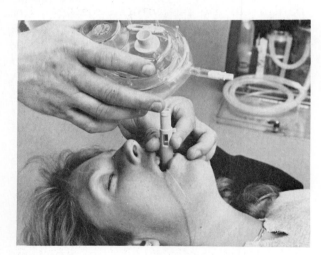

Figure 2.63.

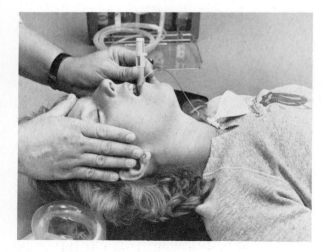

Figure 2.64.

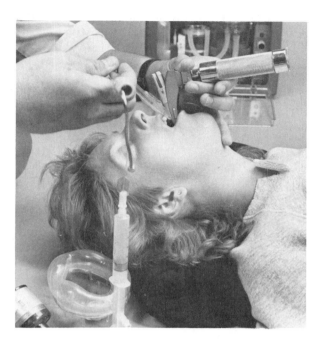

Figure 2.65.

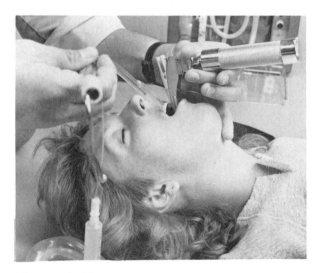

Figure 2.66.

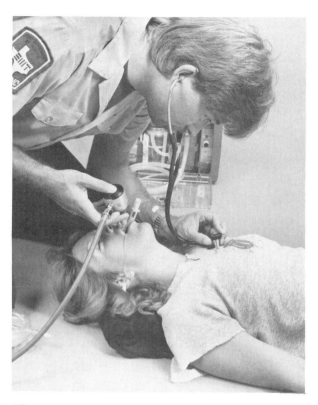

Figure 2.67.

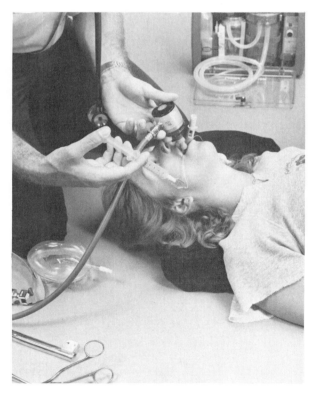

Figure 2.68.

Insert the laryngoscope, and visualize the laryngeal opening (Figure 2.65).

Insert the endotracheal tube (Figure 2.66).

Check tube placement by auscultating the chest and watching for it to rise (Figure 2.67).

Inflate the cuff (Figure 2.68). You must check the pulse again at this point. A few cases have been reported where

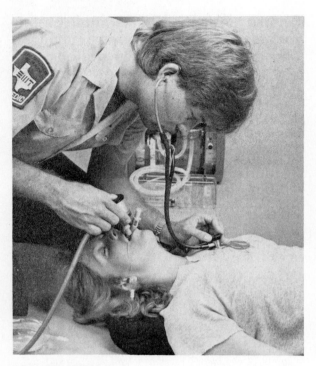

Figure 2.69.

concurrent inflation of both the EOA and ET cuffs have created enough pressure to stimulate the vagus nerves, thus causing a slowing or arrest of the heart.

Auscultate the lungs (Figure 2.69).

Removal of EOA

While maintaining ventilation, turn the patient's head to the side (if C-spine injury has been ruled out) (Figure 2.70).

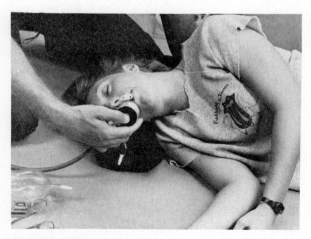

Figure 2.70.

Insert the suction catheter and deflate the EOA cuff (Figure 2.71).

Remove the EOA tube while maintaining suction (Figure 2.72).

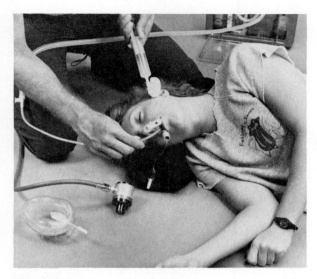

Figure 2.71.

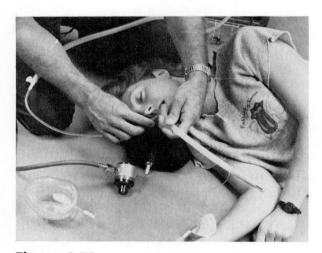

Figure 2.72.

STUDENT NAME _____ **DATE** _____

DIRECTIONS

Evaluate the student by using the criteria presented on this form. Mark PASS for an appropriate action. Mark FAIL for an inappropriate action or missed step. An asterisk (*) indicates an absolute step. Omission of this step indicates automatic failure.

	STEP	PASS	FAIL
1.	Tests cuff on endotracheal tube*	[ ]	[ ]
2.	Checks laryngoscope and light*	[ ]	[ ]
3.	Chooses an appropriate blade	[ ]	[ ]
4.	Maintains ventilation with EOA	[ ]	[ ]
5.	Hyperventilates patient*	[ ]	[ ]
6.	Removes EOA mask*	[ ]	[ ]
7.	Moves EOA tube to left side of mouth	[ ]	[ ]
8.	Inserts laryngoscope	[ ]	[ ]
9.	Visualizes cords*	[ ]	[ ]
10.	Inserts endotracheal tube while maintaining visualization of cords	[ ]	[ ]
11.	Checks tube placement*	[ ]	[ ]
12.	Inflates cuff	[ ]	[ ]
13.	Auscultates lungs and abdomen*	[ ]	[ ]
14.	Completes steps 6-11 in 20 seconds or less*	[ ]	[ ]
15.	While maintaining ventilation turns patient head to side	[ ]	[ ]
16.	Inserts suction catheter	[ ]	[ ]
17.	Deflates EOA cuff*	[ ]	[ ]
18.	Removes EOA	[ ]	[ ]
19.	Maintains suction	[ ]	[ ]
20.	Reassesses airway*	[ ]	[ ]

TOTAL SCORE (2 points for each PASS) _____
(35 required for PASS)
NO ABSOLUTES MAY BE FAILED

_____ _____
Evaluator   Date

Nasotracheal Intubation

Overview

Nasotracheal intubation is the placement of an endotracheal tube through the nose into the trachea. Nasotracheal intubation is preferred in patients who have suffered trauma to the mouth or face. Nasotracheal intubation is not as uncomfortable to the patient as orotracheal intubation and is often preferred when long-term airway management is required.

Indications

1. Patients in deep coma, respiratory arrest, or cardiopulmonary arrest, especially where trauma to the face or mouth is apparent.
2. Patients where long-term intubation may be indicated.

Contraindications

Same as orotracheal intubation.

Precautions

The same precautions apply to nasotracheal intubation as apply to orotracheal intubation. A stylet is not required because of the technique employed in nasotracheal intubation.

If a basal skull fracture is suspected, nasotracheal intubation is best deferred until the patient is in the emergency department. If the skull fracture communicates with the nasopharynx, as occasionally happens, attempting to intubate via this route can result in the endotracheal tube being forced into the cranial vault through the fracture. The results can, of course, be disastrous.

Complications

Same as orotracheal intubation.

Required Equipment

- Endotracheal tube
- Lubricant
- 10-mL syringe
- McGill forceps
- Laryngoscope blade
- Laryngoscope handle
- 1-inch Adhesive tape

Procedure

PREPARE AND CHECK EQUIPMENT

Test the cuff and apply water-soluble lubricant to end of tube (Figure 2.73).

Prepare equipment (Figure 2.74).

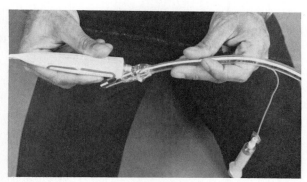

Figure 2.73.

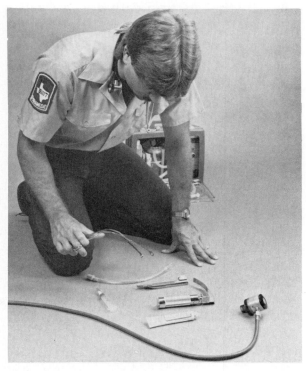

Figure 2.74.

Inspect the nose to determine whether there is any septal deviation, mucosal hypertrophy, or any other factors which render one side more patent than the other (Figure 2.75).

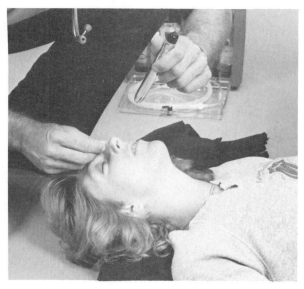

Figure 2.75.

INTUBATION PROCEDURE

Hyperventilate the patient (Figure 2.76).

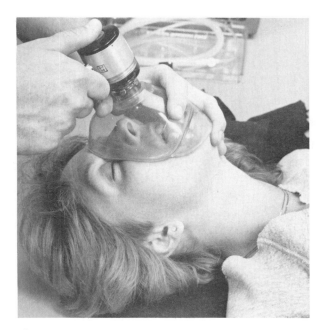

Figure 2.76.

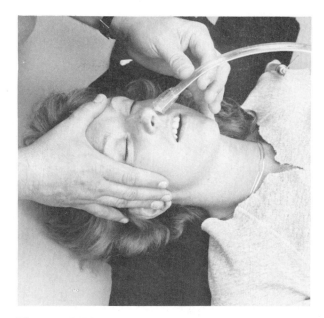

Figure 2.77.

Maintain the patient's head in a neutral position and insert the lubricated endotracheal tube into the nose (Figure 2.77).

Advance the endotracheal tube to where it is in the floor of the oropharynx (Figure 2.78).

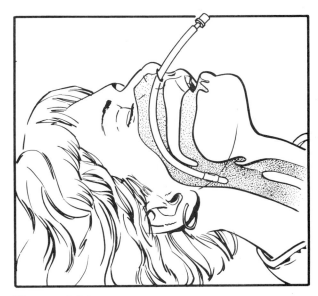

Figure 2.78.

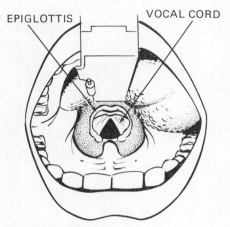

Figure 2.79.

Visualize the larynx with the laryngoscope (Figure 2.79).

Grasp the end of the endotracheal tube with the McGill forceps and advance the tube into the glottic opening (Figure 2.80). Maintain visualization as the tube is inserted.

Check tube placement (Figure 2.81).

Inflate the cuff, and auscultate the lungs (Figure 2.82).

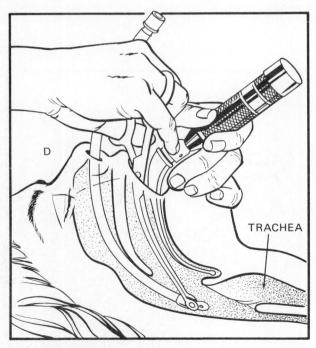

Figure 2.80.

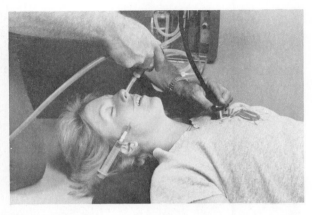

Figure 2.81.

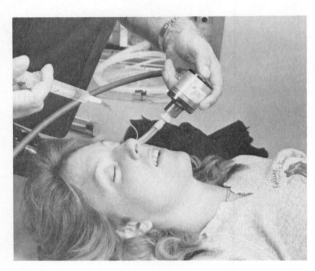

Figure 2.82.

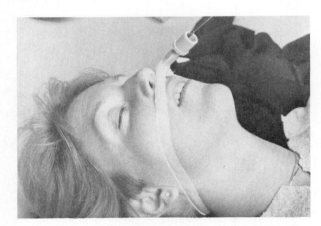

Figure 2.83.

Anchor the tube to the face with adhesive tape (Figure 2.83).

STUDENT NAME _____ **DATE** _____

DIRECTIONS

Evaluate the student by using the criteria presented on this form. Mark PASS for an appropriate action. Mark FAIL for an inappropriate action or missed step. An asterisk (*) indicates an absolute step. Omission of this step indicates automatic failure.

	STEP	PASS	FAIL
1.	Tests cuff*	[ ]	[ ]
2.	Checks laryngoscope and light*	[ ]	[ ]
3.	Selects appropriate tube*	[ ]	[ ]
4.	Applies lubricant to tube	[ ]	[ ]
5.	Inspects nose and selects side	[ ]	[ ]
6.	Hyperventilates patient*	[ ]	[ ]
7.	Inserts tube in nose	[ ]	[ ]
8.	Advances tube to oropharynx	[ ]	[ ]
9.	Inserts laryngoscope properly	[ ]	[ ]
10.	Visualizes airway and vocal cords*	[ ]	[ ]
11.	Inserts McGill forceps	[ ]	[ ]
12.	Grasps tube and inserts through glottic opening	[ ]	[ ]
13.	Checks tube placement*	[ ]	[ ]
14.	Ventilates patient*	[ ]	[ ]
15.	Auscultates chest*	[ ]	[ ]
16.	Secures tube properly	[ ]	[ ]
17.	Performs steps 7-13 in 25 seconds or less*	[ ]	[ ]
18.	Reassesses airway	[ ]	[ ]

TOTAL SCORE (2 points for each PASS) _____
(26 required for PASS)
NO ABSOLUTES MAY BE FAILED

_____   _____
            Evaluator   Date

Blind Nasotracheal Intubation

Overview

Blind nasotracheal intubation is rarely used in the prehospital setting. Like all of the other airway management skills discussed thus far, blind nasotracheal intubation requires considerable skill, which can only be obtained after considerable supervised practice.

Blind intubation is used to place endotracheal tubes in patients who are still breathing and who may often be conscious. This is sometimes necessary in managing patients who have suffered a drug overdose or in patients who suffer injuries or illnesses that seriously impair their ability to adequately maintain their own airway or adequately ventilate.

Indications

Patients who are still breathing yet who are unable to adequately manage their own airway. **This technique is not frequently indicated in prehospital care.**

Contraindications

Same as orotracheal intubation.

Precautions

Failure to clear the airway prior to starting this procedure may result in foreign material being accidentally forced into the trachea from the oropharynx.

The most common problem with this procedure is the accidental introduction of the endotracheal tube into the esophagus. Occasionally the tip of the tube may become lodged in the vallecula. Anterior displacement of the mandible often relieves this problem.

Complications

1. Accidental intubation of the esophagus.

2. Insertion of the endotracheal tube too far (endobronchial intubation).
3. Oropharyngeal and laryngopharyngeal trauma.
4. Spasm of the vocal cords.

Required Equipment

- Endotracheal tube
- 10-mL Syringe
- Lubricant
- 1-inch Adhesive tape

Procedure

PREPARE AND CHECK EQUIPMENT

Test the cuff on the endotracheal tube and apply water-soluble lubricant (Figure 2.84).

INTUBATION PROCEDURE

Inspect the nose to determine whether there is any septal deviation, mucosal hypertrophy, or any other factors which render one side more patent than the other (Figure 2.85).

Place the patient's head in a neutral position, and insert the endotracheal tube through the nose and into the oropharynx (Figure 2.86).

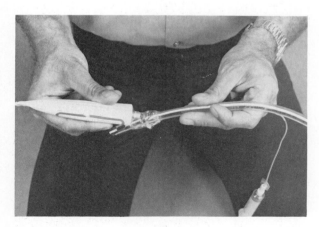

Figure 2.84.

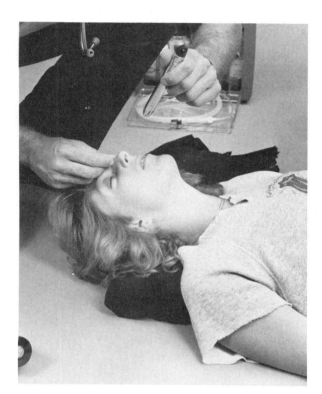

Figure 2.85.

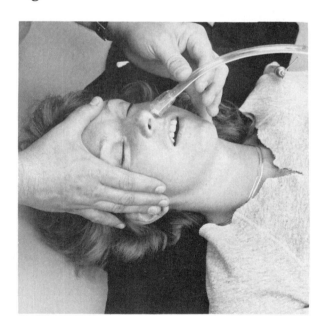

Figure 2.86.

Advance the tube while listening for respiratory sounds over the tube. When these are heard, the tube is at the glottic opening (Figure 2.87).

Advance the tube through the glottis **During Inspiration** with a single rapid movement (Figure 2.88). Listen for the passage of air, which indicates correct placement. If there is no passage of air, the tube is probably in the esophagus and should be removed.

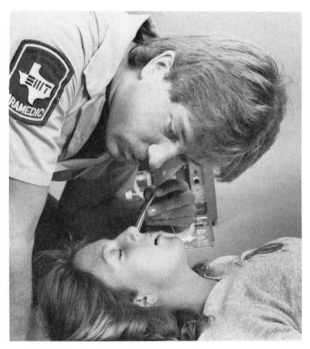

Figure 2.87.

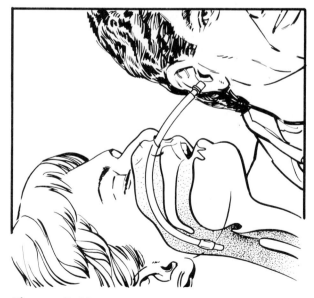

Figure 2.88.

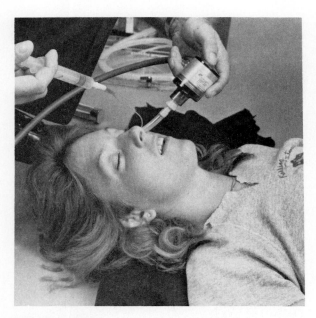

Figure 2.89.

Inflate the cuff and secure the tube (Figure 2.89).

Tracheal Suctioning

Overview

Tracheal suctioning may be required to clear secretions from the airway. It is generally performed through the endotracheal tube and must be done quite rapidly to avoid depriving the patient of air. Prior to beginning tracheal suctioning, the patient should be ventilated with oxygen to elevate circulating oxygen levels. In addition, sterile technique is required to reduce the chances of inducing a pulmonary infection.

Indications

Tracheal suctioning is indicated in patients with noisy respirations and with an endotracheal tube in place.

Contraindications

Tracheal suctioning is not without danger and should be performed only when the airway is compromised by secretions or aspirated material.

Precautions

Tracheal suctioning should never last more than 10 seconds. Prolonged tracheal suctioning will produce hypoxia and may cause vagally mediated dysrhythmias. Cardiac arrest from tracheal suctioning has been reported. Prior to beginning tracheal suctioning the patient should be well oxygenated. Trauma to the trachea, including hemorrhage, can result from repeated tracheal suctioning. The suction catheter should always have a side thumb vent, and its external diameter should be no larger than one-third the size of the endotracheal tube.

If possible, the patient should be placed on a cardiac monitor before beginning this procedure.

Complications

1. Hypoxia and cardiac dysrhythmias
2. Tracheal and oropharyngeal trauma
3. Pulmonary infection

Required Equipment

- Sterile catheter
- Sterile rinse solution
- Sterile glove
- Suction device

Procedure

PREPARE EQUIPMENT   Figure 2.90 shows the suction catheter kit.

To begin the suctioning procedure, put on sterile gloves (Figure 2.91). With the increasing incidence of herpes virus infections (both type I and II), double gloving (two gloves on each hand) is often recommended.

SUCTIONING PROCEDURE   Grasp the catheter with the gloved hand (Figure 2.92).

Inset the catheter into the trachea (Figure 2.93).

Cover the thumb vent to begin suctioning (Figure 2.94).

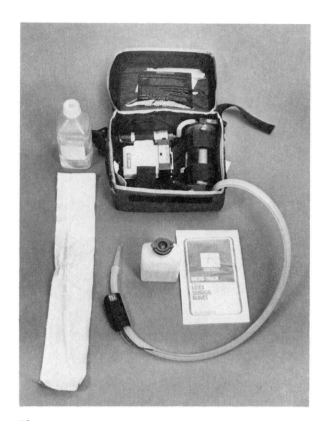

Figure 2.90.

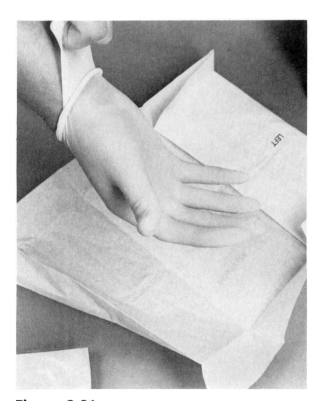

Figure 2.91.

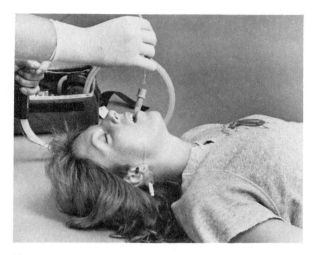

Figure 2.92.

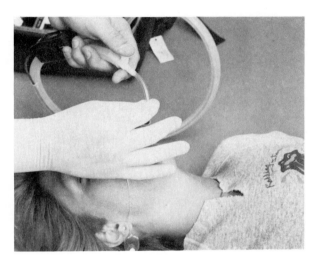

Figure 2.93.

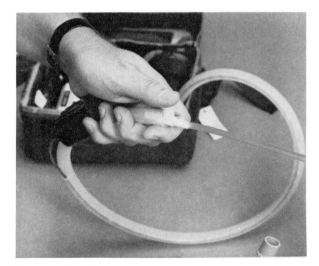

Figure 2.94.

Remove the catheter, by maintaining suctioning and rotating the catheter (Figure 2.95).

Rinse the catheter in a sterile solution if more suctioning is required (Figure 2.96). However, do not immediately re-suction.

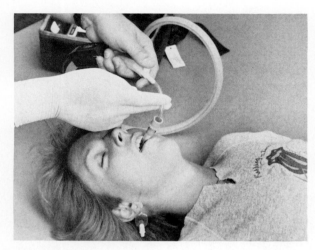

Figure 2.95.

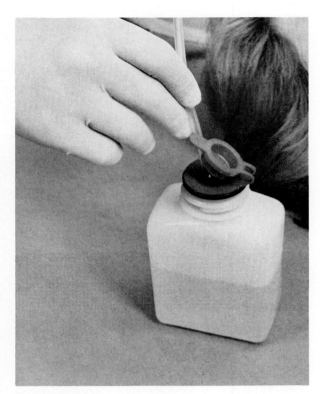

Figure 2.96.

STUDENT NAME _____ **DATE** _____

DIRECTIONS

Evaluate the student by using the criteria presented on this form. Mark PASS for an appropriate action. Mark FAIL for an inappropriate action or missed step. An asterisk (*) indicates an absolute step. Omission of this step indicates automatic failure.

STEP	PASS	FAIL
1. Prepares equipment	[ ]	[ ]
2. Dons sterile gloves	[ ]	[ ]
3. Grasps suction catheter with gloved hand	[ ]	[ ]
4. Interrupts ventilation	[ ]	[ ]
5. Inserts suction catheter	[ ]	[ ]
6. Applies suction as tube is withdrawn	[ ]	[ ]
7. Does not suction for longer than 10 seconds*	[ ]	[ ]
8. Removes and rinses catheter	[ ]	[ ]
9. Reventilates patient*	[ ]	[ ]
10. Reassesses airway	[ ]	[ ]

TOTAL SCORE (2 points for each PASS) _____
(14 required for PASS)
NO ABSOLUTES MAY BE FAILED

_____   _____
            Evaluator   Date

Airway Clearance with McGill Forceps

Overview

Direct visualization of the airway via laryngoscopy provides a method for removing an airway obstruction when other manual methods, such as the Heimlich manuever, fail. The glottic opening is visualized in much the same manner as for endotracheal intubation. However, when the obstructing body is located, and if it is within reach of the McGill forceps, it is removed. Often, airway obstructions are not found until endotracheal intubation is attempted.

Indications

Airway obstructions that cannot be removed by other procedures.

Contraindications

This procedure is only effective on obstructions that can be reached with the McGill forceps and on non-anatomical obstructions.

Precautions

Avoid touching vocal cords during this procedure to avoid inducing vocal cord spasm. Also, it is easy to accidently grab a portion of the patient's airway (i.e., tongue, pharnygeal wall, or laryngeal structures) if not cautious.

Complications

1. Spasm of the vocal cords
2. Trauma to the pharynx and/or larynx
3. Hemorrhage

Required Equipment

- McGill forceps
- Laryngoscope handle
- Laryngoscope blade
- suction

Procedure

Confirm airway obstruction. Attempt Heimlich or similar maneuver (Figure 2.97).

Hyperextend the patient's neck, and visualize the larynx (Figure 2.98).

Insert the McGill forceps (Figure 2.99).

Grasp the airway obstruction, and gently remove it (Figure 2.100).

Reassess the airway status (Figure 2.101). Administer supplemental oxygen.

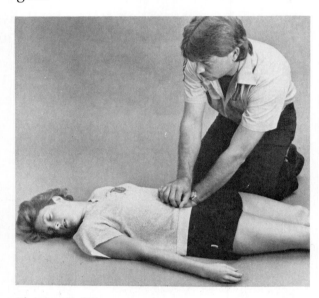

Figure 2.97.

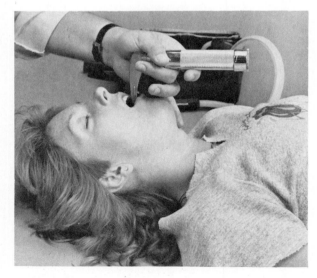

Figure 2.98.

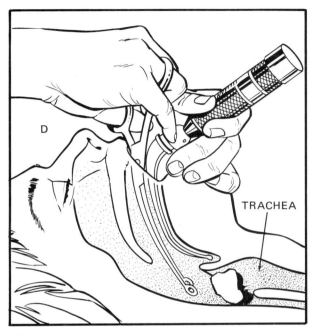

Figure 2.99.

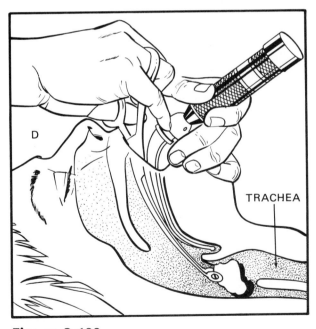

Figure 2.100.

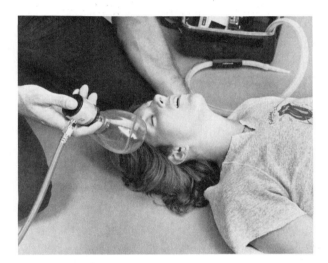

Figure 2.101.

STUDENT NAME _____ **DATE** _____

DIRECTIONS

Evaluate the student by using the criteria presented on this form. Mark PASS for an appropriate action. Mark FAIL for an inappropriate action or missed step. An asterisk (*) indicates an absolute step. Omission of this step indicates automatic failure.

STEP	PASS	FAIL
1. Confirm airway obstruction* and reattempt BLS procedures	[ ]	[ ]
2. Prepare equipment	[ ]	[ ]
3. Hyperextend neck	[ ]	[ ]
4. Insert laryngoscope and visualize glottic opening	[ ]	[ ]
5. Identify obstruction	[ ]	[ ]
6. Insert McGill forceps	[ ]	[ ]
7. Grasp obstruction and remove	[ ]	[ ]
8. Remove laryngoscope	[ ]	[ ]
9. Reassess airway*	[ ]	[ ]
10. Document removal on patient report	[ ]	[ ]

TOTAL SCORE (2 points for each PASS)   _____
(14 required for PASS)
NO ABSOLUTES MAY BE FAILED

_____   _____
              Evaluator   Date

Surgical Cricothyrotomy

Overview

Surgical cricothyrotomy is an invasive skill reserved for cases of airway obstruction that fail to respond to all other techniques. Surgical cricothyrotomy is a surgical opening of the trachea, through the cricothyroid membrane, to effect ventilation.

Several commercial devices are available and are preferred for performing cricothyrotomy in the prehospital setting. These devices do not require an incision and can be inserted in a one-step fashion.
This Procedure is Rarely Indicated in Prehospital Care.

Indications

1.   Complete airway obstruction that cannot be cleared by manual techniques or by direct visualization via laryngoscopy.
2.   Occasional cases of SEVERE facial trauma that make the use of any adjunctive airway device impossible.

Contraindications

Surgical cricothyrotomy should only be employed in life-threatening cases of airway obstruction where the obstruction cannot be cleared by any other means.

Precautions

The paramedic must follow the procedure exactly and must pay particular attention to finding the cricothyroid membrane. If possible, this procedure should be practiced on a cadaver or on a laboratory animal.

Several arteries and nerves are located in the anterior portion of the neck. Accidental injury to these structures, including moderate hemorrhage, is possible.

Complications

1.   Hemorrhage
2.   Injury to the thyroid or parathyroid glands.
3.   Damage to the larynx
4.   False passage
5.   Subcutaneous and mediastinal emphysema

Required Equipment

- Scalpel
- Tracheotomy tube
- Sponges
- Skin retractor
- Bacteriocidal prep
- 10-mL Syringe
- Hemostats

Procedure

Figure 2.102 shows a cricothyroidotomy kit.

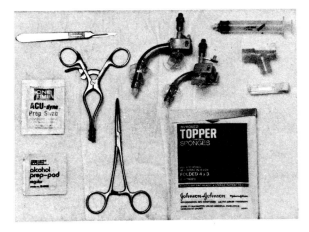

Figure 2.102.

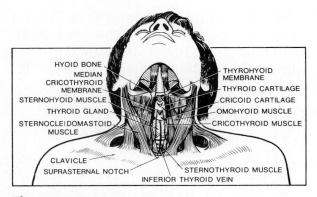

Figure 2.103.

The anatomy of the cricothyroid membrane is show in Figure 2.103.

A front view of the larynx is shown in Figure 2.104.

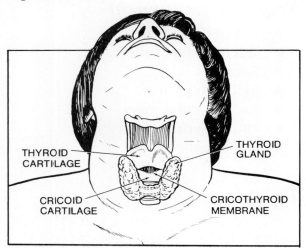

Figure 2.104.

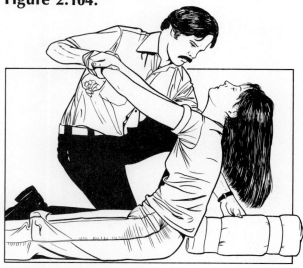

Figure 2.105.

Hyperextend the patient's neck (if no C-spine injury is suspected (Figure 2.105).

Identify the cricothyroid membrane (Figure 2.106).

Prepare the skin by scrubbing with an antibacterial solution (Figure 2.107).

Incise the skin over the cricothyroid membrane; be careful not to penetrate too deeply (Figure 2.108).

Apply a skin retractor (Figure 2.109).

Incise cricothyroid membrane (Figure 2.110).

Enlarge the opening (Figure 2.111).

Insert the tracheotomy tube (Figure 2.112).

Remove the stylus (Figure 2.113).

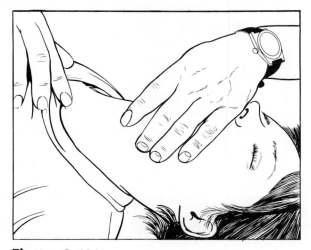

Figure 2.106.

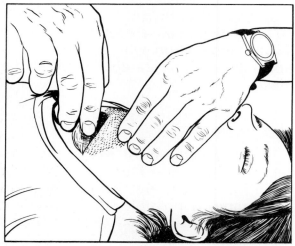

Figure 2.107.

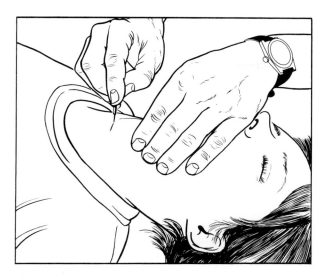

Figure 2.108.

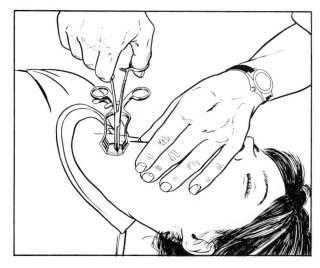

Figure 2.111.

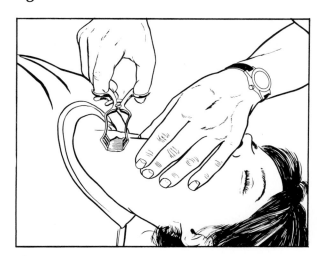

Figure 2.109.

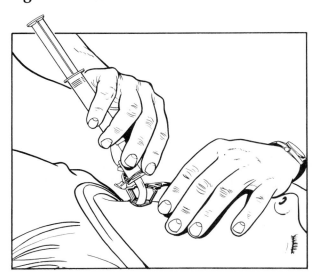

Figure 2.112.

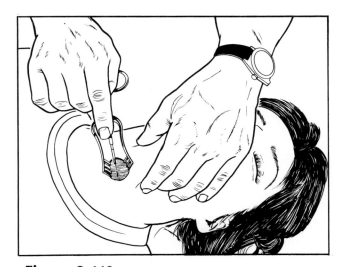

Figure 2.110.

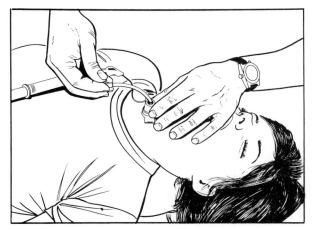

Figure 2.113.

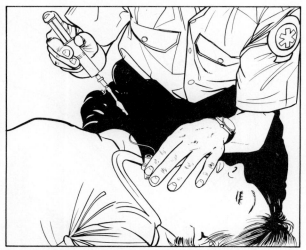

Figure 2.114.

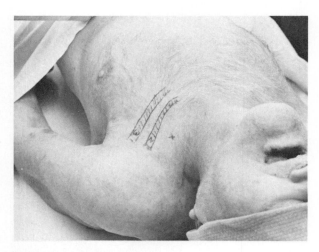

Figure 2.116.

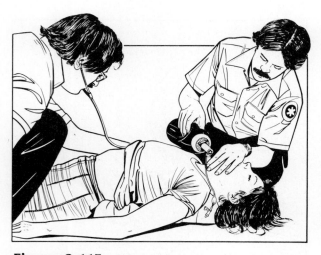

Figure 2.115.

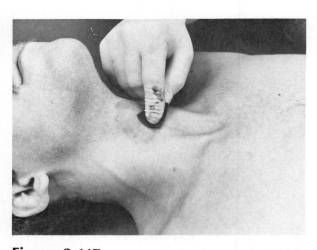

Figure 2.117.

Inflate the cuff (Figure 2.114).
Ventilate and auscultate (Figure 2.115).

Alternate Technique

Extend the patient's neck, and palpate the cricothyroid membrane (Figure 2.116).

Prep the skin over the membrane if time permits (Figure 2.117).

Puncture the skin and membrane with a 14-gauge, indwelling IV catheter or commercial cricothyrotomy device (Figure 2.118).

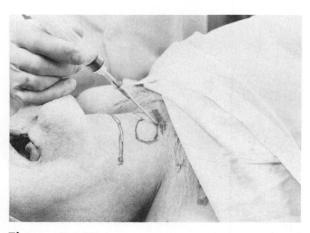

Figure 2.118.

Remove the stylet (Figure 2.119).
Place the oxygen mask over the catheter (Figure 2.120).
If necessary, ventilate with a syringe (Figure 2.121).

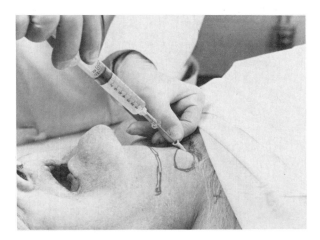

Figure 2.119.

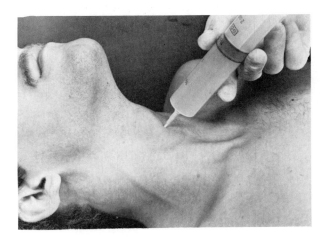

Figure 2.121.

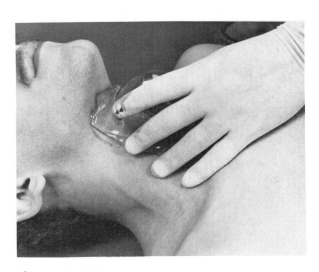

Figure 2.120.

STUDENT NAME _____ **DATE** _____

DIRECTIONS

Evaluate the student by using the criteria presented on this form. Mark PASS for an appropriate action. Mark FAIL for an inappropriate action or missed step. An asterisk (*) indicates an absolute step. Omission of this step indicates automatic failure.

STEP	PASS	FAIL
1. Explains indications for this skill*	[ ]	[ ]
2. Prepares supplies	[ ]	[ ]
3. Hyperextends the neck	[ ]	[ ]
4. Identifies cricothyroid membrane*	[ ]	[ ]
5. Preps skin	[ ]	[ ]
6. Incises skin over membrane	[ ]	[ ]
7. Applies skin retractor	[ ]	[ ]
8. Incises cricothyroid membrane	[ ]	[ ]
9. Enlarges the opening	[ ]	[ ]
10. Inserts tracheotomy tube	[ ]	[ ]
11. Removes stylus	[ ]	[ ]
12. Inflates the cuff	[ ]	[ ]
13. Ventilates and auscultates*	[ ]	[ ]

TOTAL SCORE (2 points for each PASS) _____
(20 required for PASS)
NO ABSOLUTES MAY BE FAILED

_____   _____
                Evaluator   Date

Chapter Objectives

Upon completion of this chapter, the student should be able to:

1. List the indications, contraindications, precautions, and common complications of the following procedures:

    *   Tension pneumothorax decompression with a needle
    *   Tension pneumothorax decompression with a McSwain dart

2. Be able to perform the following procedures according to the criteria presented:

    *   Tension pneumothorax decompression with a needle
    *   Tension pneumothorax decompression with a McSwain dart

3

Tension Pneumothorax Decompression Skills

Overview

Decompression of a tension pneumothorax is a prehospital skill that is used infrequently, yet it is quite important. A tension pneumothorax occurs when air is drawn into the pleural space on inspiration and is not removed with expiration (Figure 3.1). Tension pneumothorax can either result from a hole in the chest or from an internal leak of air from the lung. As air continues to fill the pleural space, the lungs and trachea are pushed to the side of the chest opposite the injury. Eventually, the lungs will be so compressed that ventilation is seriously compromised. The pressure inside the chest will exceed that of the blood pressure, and eventually blood return to the heart will be reduced. If not treated, tension pneumothorax will rapidly become fatal.

Clinically, the patient with a tension pneumothorax exhibits cyanosis, dyspnea, neck vein distension, absent breath sounds on one side of the chest, and, occasionally, tracheal deviation away from the affected side.

Tension pneumothorax is treated by placing a needle into the chest to alleviate the pressure. This procedure can be done either by insertion of a standard needle or by use of a commercial pleural decompression device such as the

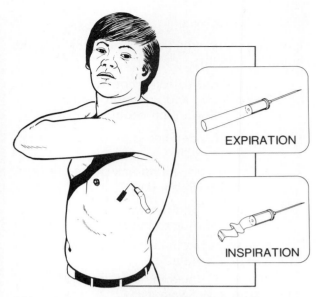

Figure 3.2. Needle decompression illustrating a one-way valve.

McSwain dart. These measures are temporary, and the needle should be replaced by a chest tube when the patient arrives at the emergency department.

The needle should be inserted into the affected side of the chest at the fourth intercostal space in a mid-axillary line. An alternate placement site is the second intercostal space in a mid-clavicular line.

The needle used for decompression should have a one-way valve attached to prevent air re-entry through the needle. Commercial devices, such as the McSwain dart, come with a one-way valve already attached. A one-way valve can be constructed from the finger of a glove (Figure 3.2.).

Puncture of the chest wall will often be accompanied by a hissing of air as the chest is decompressed and often an immediate improvement in the clinical status of the patient.

Indications

Suspected tension pneumothorax displaying dyspnea, cyanosis, shallow respirations, jugular venous distension, and tracheal deviation.

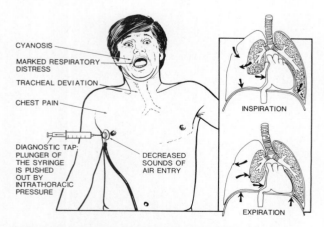

CYANOSIS

MARKED RESPIRATORY DISTRESS

TRACHEAL DEVIATION

CHEST PAIN

DIAGNOSTIC TAP: PLUNGER OF THE SYRINGE IS PUSHED OUT BY INTRATHORACIC PRESSURE

DECREASED SOUNDS OF AIR ENTRY

INSPIRATION

EXPIRATION

Figure 3.1. Tension pneumothorax.

Contraindications

None when used in the setting of tension pneumothorax.

Precautions

When making the puncture, DO NOT penetrate any further than the pleura. Quite often you will feel a "pop" as the needle is advanced through the pleura. Too deep an insertion of the needle may result in penetration of the lung. This statement is especially true in cases where the lung is not totally collapsed.

You must also make the puncture as close to the superior border of the lateral ribs as possible to avoid the intercostal artery, vein, and nerve.

Complications

1. Puncture of the lung

2. Hemorrhage from puncture of the intercostal vessels
3. Hemorrhage from puncture of a pulmonary vessel

Required Equipment

- 14-gauge Indwelling catheter or intracath
- One-way valve (or finger from glove)
- Adhesive tape
- Antibacterial prep

Procedure

DECOMPRESSION WITH NEEDLE

Cut the intracath plastic sleeve to form a one-way valve (Figure 3.3).

Remove the wire stylet (Figure 3.4).

Confirm unequal air entry (Figure 3.5).

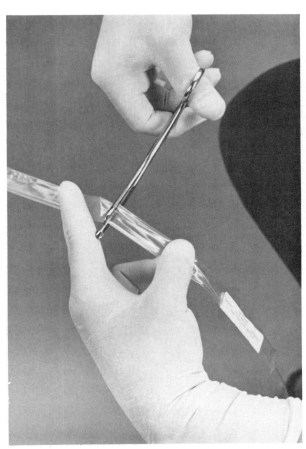

Figure 3.3.

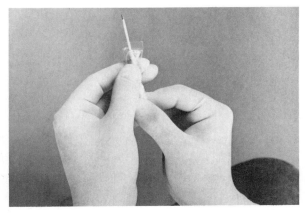

Figure 3.4.

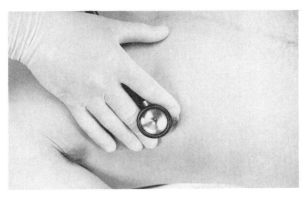

Figure 3.5.

Confirm tracheal deviation, and mark the location of the trachea with a ball-point pen (Figure 3.6).

Palpate the fourth interspace in the mid-axillary line (Figure 3.7).

Prep the site with an antibacterial solution (Figure 3.8).

Insert the needle along the superior border of the fifth rib (Figure 3.9).

Anatomy of the fourth interspace (Figure 3.10).

Check for improvement in the patient's clinical status (for example, pulse, respirations) (Figure 3.11).

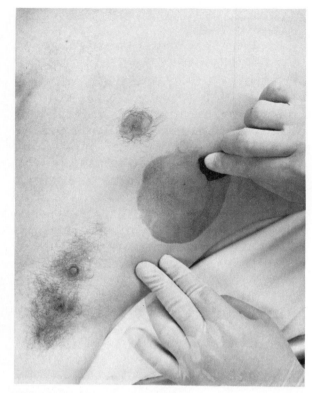

Figure 3.8.

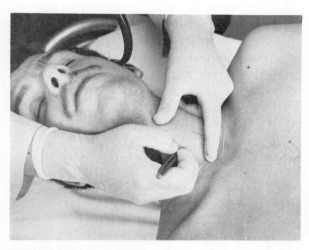

Figure 3.6.

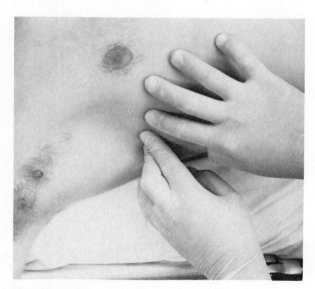

Figure 3.7.

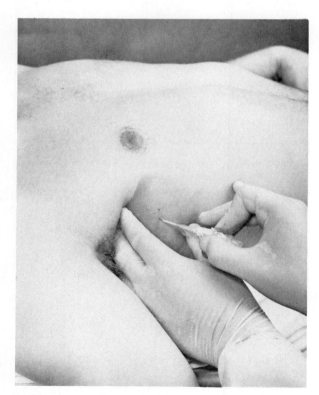

Figure 3.9.

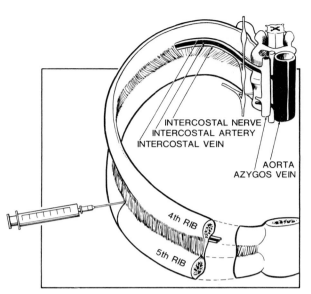

Figure 3.10.

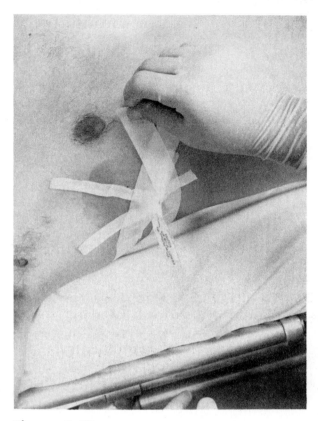

Figure 3.12.

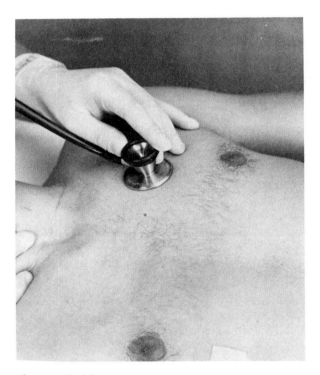

Figure 3.11.

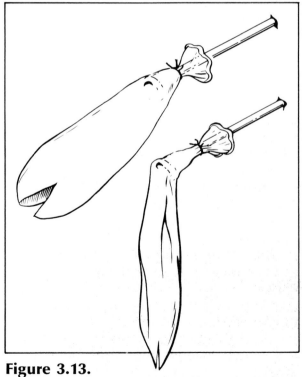

Figure 3.13.

Tape the needle in place, and assure that the flutter valve is functioning properly (Figure 3.12).

The flutter valve during expiration and inspiration is shown in Figure 3.13, A and B, respectively.

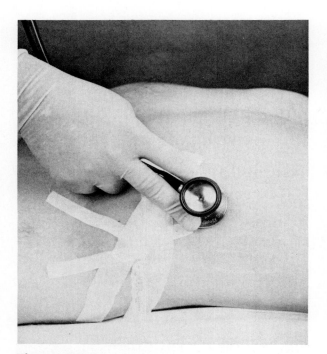

Figure 3.14.

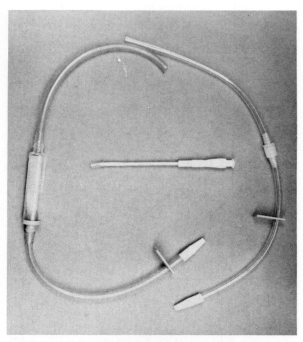

Figure 3.15. McSwain dart with valve.

Reassess air entry into the affected side (Figure 3.14).

Insertion of the McSwain Dart

REQUIRED EQUIPMENT
- McSwain dart (trocar with cannula) (Figure 3.15)
- Heimlich valve with setup
- Antibacterial prep
- Scalpel

TECHNIQUE   Identify the fourth intercostal space in a mid-axillary line (Figure 3.16).

Prepare the area with an antibacterial solution (Figure 3.17).

Make a "nick" through the skin at the superior border of the fifth rib to facilitate insertion of the trocar (Figure 3.18).

Insert the dart approximately 1 inch at a 90° angle through the "nick" (Figure 3.19).

After the pleural cavity is entered, advance the dart another 0.5 inch, and remove the stylet, and immediately attach the tubing to the Heimlich valve (Figure 3.20).

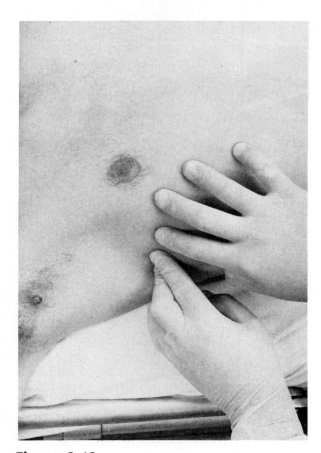

Figure 3.16.

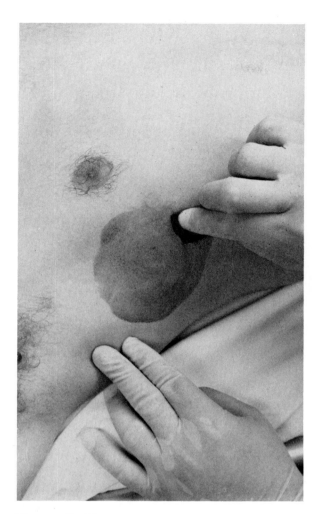

Figure 3.17.

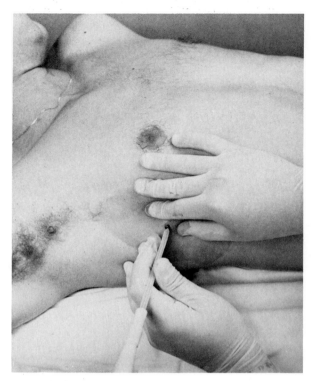

Figure 3.19.

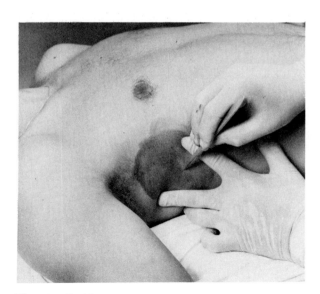

Figure 3.18.

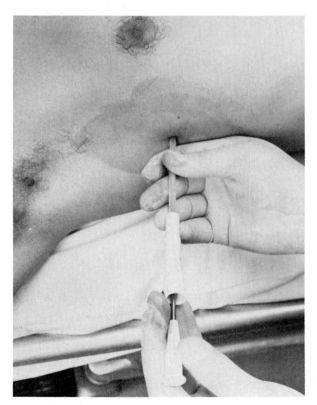

Figure 3.20.

Extend the wings of the dart by advancing the flared fittings (Figure 3.21).

Figure 3.22 shows the valve with wings flared.

Retract the device until contact with the chest wall is made (Figure 3.23).

Tape the dart in place (Figure 3.24).

Reassess the ventilation (Figure 3.25).

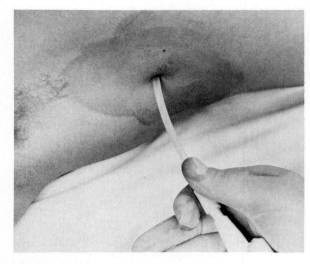

Figure 3.23.

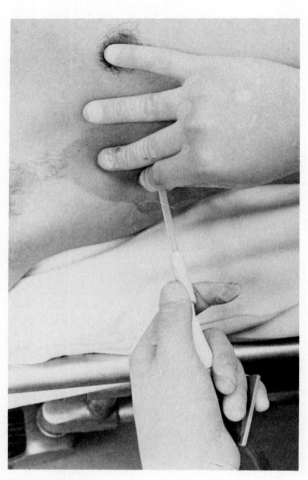

Figure 3.21.

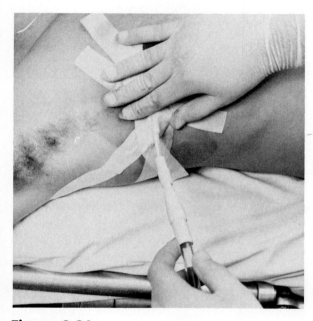

Figure 3.24.

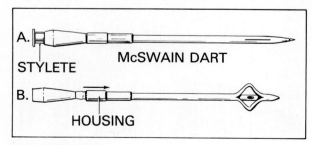

Figure 3.22.

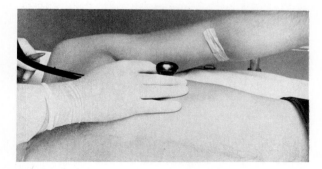

Figure 3.25.

STUDENT NAME _____ **DATE** _____

DIRECTIONS

Evaluate the student by using the criteria presented on this form. Mark PASS for an appropriate action. Mark FAIL for an inappropriate action or missed step. An asterisk (*) indicates an absolute step. Omission of this step indicates automatic failure.

STEP	PASS	FAIL
NEEDLE METHOD		
1. Understands indications*	[ ]	[ ]
2. Prepares equipment	[ ]	[ ]
3. Confirms unequal air entry*	[ ]	[ ]
4. Palpates 4th interspace at mid-axillary line	[ ]	[ ]
5. Preps site	[ ]	[ ]
6. Inserts needle at superior border of 5th rib*	[ ]	[ ]
7. Checks for improvement in clinical status	[ ]	[ ]
8. Checks flutter valve	[ ]	[ ]
9. Tapes needle in place	[ ]	[ ]
10. Reassesses ventilations*	[ ]	[ ]
McSWAIN DART INSERTION		
1. Understands indications*	[ ]	[ ]
2. Prepares equipment	[ ]	[ ]
3. Confirms unequal air entry*	[ ]	[ ]
4. Palpates 4th interspace at mid-axillary line.	[ ]	[ ]
5. Preps site	[ ]	[ ]
6. Inserts the dart at the superior border of the 5th rib*	[ ]	[ ]
7. Enters additional ½ inch after puncturing the pleural cavity.	[ ]	[ ]
8. Attaches the Heimlich valve and extends wings of dart	[ ]	[ ]
9. Retracts valve and tapes in place	[ ]	[ ]
10. Reassesses ventilations	[ ]	[ ]

TOTAL SCORE (2 points for each PASS) _____
(14 required for PASS)
NO ABSOLUTES MAY BE FAILED

_____   _____
Evaluator   Date

Chapter Objectives

Upon completion of this chapter, the student should be able to:

1. List the indications, contraindications, precautions, and common complications of the following procedures:

   - Adult anti-shock trouser application
   - Application of the mechanical CPR device
   - Insertion of an indwelling intravenous cannula

2. Be able to perform the following procedures according to the criteria presented:

   - Adult anti-shock trouser application
   - Application of the mechanical CPR device
   - Insertion of an indwelling intravenous cannula

4

Circulatory Skills

Application of the Anti-Shock Trousers (MAST)

Overview

Anti-shock trousers are a three chambered garment that can be placed over the lower extremities and abdomen to decrease blood flow to these areas which therefore shunts blood flow to such vital organs as the heart and brain. They are currently receiving widespread use in both prehospital and inhospital care for the management of hypovolemic and other forms of shock.

The anti-shock trouser was invented in 1909 by George W. Crile in conjunction with his research on hemorrhagic shock. However, the anti-shock trouser did not receive extensive clinical use until the war in Vietnam. Finally, in the early 1970s the anti-shock trouser was introduced for use in civilian prehospital care. Its efficacy has been repeatedly documented.

For many years anti-shock trousers were believed to provide a significant autotransfusion of blood from the lower extremities to the trunk. However, recent research has shown that the amount of blood autotransfused is minimal (approximately 300 mL in a 70-kg man).

Thus, anti-shock trousers are effective in combating hypovolemic shock because they significantly increase peripheral vascular resistance which serves to maintain the blood in the central portion of the body.

In addition, anti-shock trousers have proven effective in stabilizing fractures of the lower extremities. They also are receiving some use in the management of cardiac arrest where there is significant peripheral vascular collapse, which makes placement of an IV cannula difficult.

Indications

1. Hypovolemia as evidenced by a systolic pressure of less than 80 mmHg.

   Note—It is often prudent to go ahead and apply the anti-shock trousers without inflating them in patients whom you suspect might develop hypovolemic shock. This can save a great deal of time should this complication develop.

2. Fractures of the lower extremities where the anti-shock trouser may provide better stabilization than other types of splints (for example, multiple fractures).

3. Cardiac arrest where peripheral vascular collapse makes placing an IV cannula difficult.

Contraindications

The only absolute contraindication to the use of anti-shock trousers is the presence of pulmonary edema. The other contraindications to the use of the anti-shock trouser are, at present, a controversial topic. Some authorities feel that there are no contraindications when used in the management of life-threatening hypovolemic shock. Others feel there are no contraindications to the use of the suit per se, yet feel the abdominal compartment should not be inflated in cases of pregnancy beyond the second trimester and evisceration and/or impalement of the abdomen. Finally, some authorities feel that anti-shock trousers should not be used in cases of trauma above the diaphragm including head injury and chest trauma. Because of this controversy, paramedics are urged to consult their regional medical director for contraindications.

Precautions

Cases have been reported where inflation of the anti-shock trousers has resulted in a decreased capacity to effectively ventilate the lungs. This may be due to the upward pressure on the diaphragm or from direct pressure on the lower chest if the trousers are incorrectly placed. Thus, it is essential to constantly monitor the respiratory status both before and after anti-shock trouser application.

In cases of cardiac arrest, CPR should not be interrupted for more than 5 seconds while applying the trousers.

It is ESSENTIAL that the anti-shock trousers not be removed until the patient has received adequate fluid resuscitation or has been taken to the operating room for definitive treatment. **Field removal of the anti-shock trousers is absolutely contraindicated.**

Complications

1. Impaired respiratory function
2. Compartment syndrome of the lower extremities
3. Damage to abdominal organs

Procedure

APPLICATION OF THE ANTI-SHOCK TROUSERS   The anti-shock trousers are shown in Figure 4.1.

Prepare the pants by opening onto a backboard (Figure 4.2).

Pull the pants under the patient (Figure 4.3).

Position the patient (Figure 4.4).

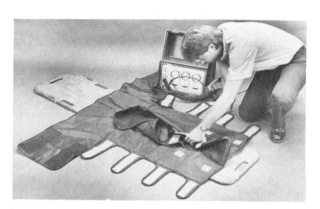

Figure 4.2.

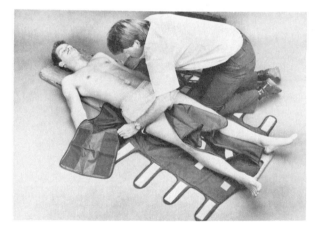

Figure 4.3.

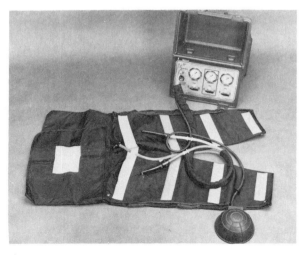

Figure 4.1.

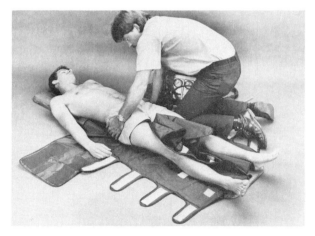

Figure 4.4.

Snugly wrap the legs and seal the Velcro connections (Figure 4.5).

Snugly close the abdominal compartment (Figure 4.6).

Connect the inflation tubes (Figure 4.7).

Close the abdominal valve, and inflate the legs first (Figure 4.8).

Inflate the trousers while monitoring the blood pressure (Figure 4.9).

Open the valve, and inflate the abdominal compartment (Figure 4.10).

Check the vital signs (Figure 4.11).

Check the pedal pulses (Figure 4.12).

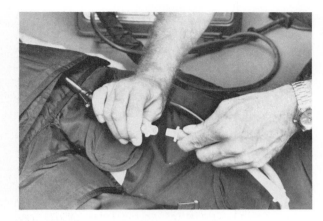

Figure 4.7.

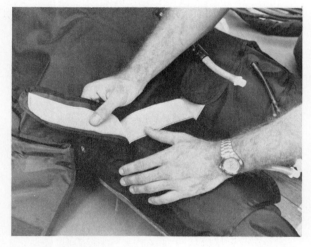

Figure 4.5.

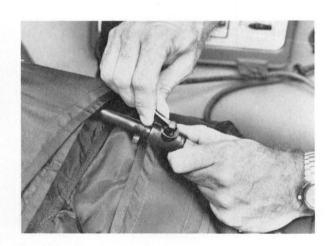

Figure 4.8.

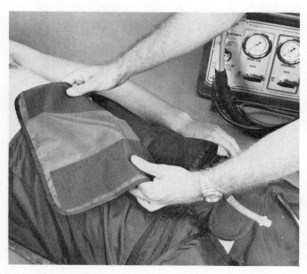

Figure 4.6.

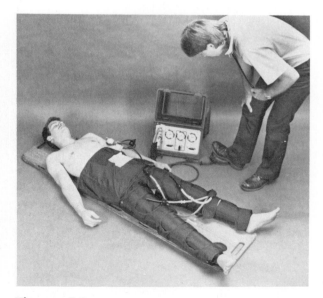

Figure 4.9.

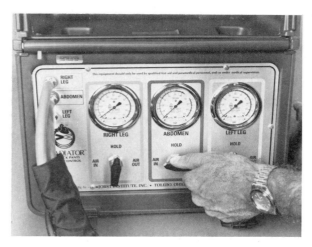

Figure 4.10.

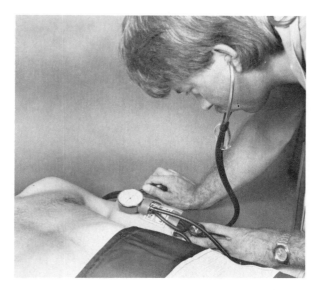

Figure 4.11.

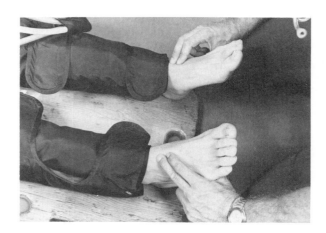

Figure 4.12.

ALTERNATE TECHNIQUE ("FAST SUIT")   An alternate technique is to have both the leg and abdominal compartments already connected (Figure 4.13).

Simply slide the anti-shock trouser onto the patient (Figure 4.14). This technique should not be used if there is a suspected injury to the lower extremities.

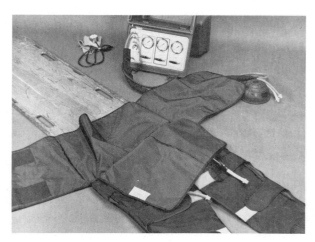

Figure 4.13.

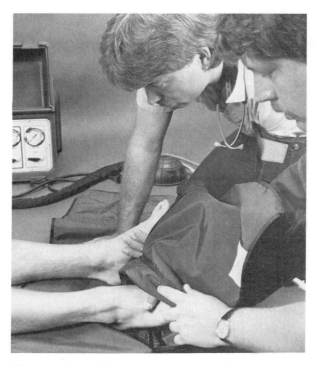

Figure 4.14.

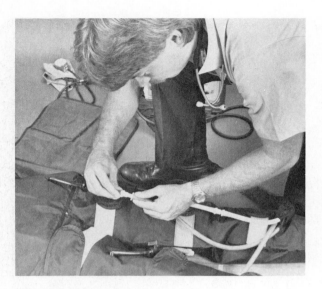

Figure 4.15.

Attach the inflation lines (Figure 4.15), and inflate as previously illustrated.

APPLICATION OF THE GAUGED ANTI-SHOCK TROUSERS   The gauged anti-shock trousers are identical to the ungauged trousers with the exception of gauges for each of the compartments which indicate intracompartmental pressure (Figure 4.16). The application of the trousers is identical. However, it is important to monitor the gauges instead of the Velcro fasteners. Also, the flow of air is controlled by a single valve instead of three.

REMOVAL OF THE ANTI-SHOCK TROUSERS   As mentioned previously, removal of the anti-shock trousers should not be attempted in the field. However, paramedics may be called upon to remove them for the emergency department staff and should be familiar with the technique.

Fluid replacement must be continued as the trousers are being slowly deflated. Generally, as the blood pressure drops 5 mmHg, deflation of the trousers is stopped, and an adequate amount of fluid is infused to increase the systolic pressure to its original value.

Monitor the blood pressure and leave BP cuff in place (Figure 4.17). You must assure that fluid resuscitation is complete.

SLOWLY release pressure in the abdominal compartment only (Figure 4.18). Release a little pressure, and then recheck the blood pressure.

Continue releasing abdominal pressure as the physical condition of the patient permits (Figure 4.19). Be prepared to reinflate the trousers or to increase the delivery of fluid if the blood pressure starts to fall. (Generally a 5 mmHg fall in the blood pressure requires the addition of more fluid.)

After all of the pressure has been released from the abdominal compartment, then begin to release pressure from one leg compartment (Figure 4.20).

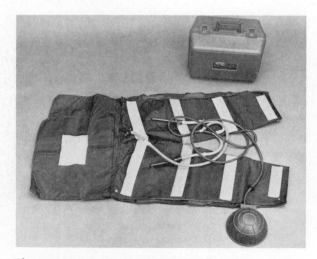

Figure 4.16. Gauged anti-shock trouser.

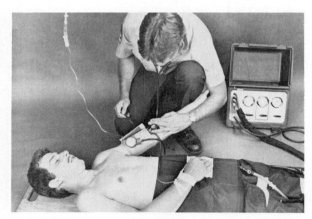

Figure 4.17.

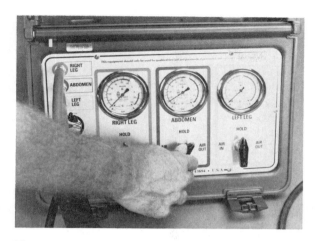

Figure 4.18.

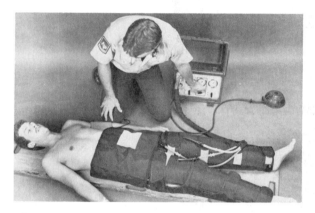

Figure 4.19.

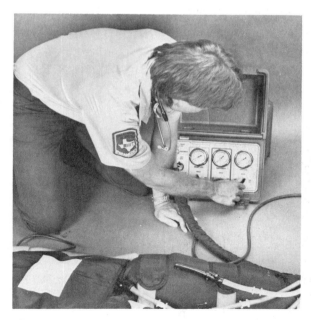

Figure 4.20.

Again, monitor the blood pressure.

After the pressure in one leg has been released, then begin to release pressure in the other leg (Figure 4.21).

After the trousers have been completely deflated, allow them to remain on the patient for at least 30 minutes in case the blood pressure again falls (Figure 4.22).

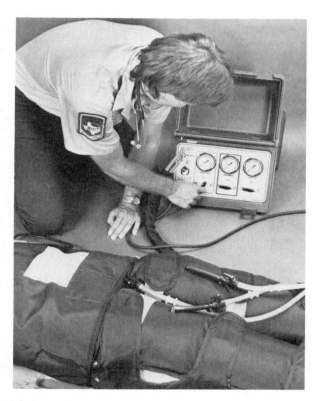

Figure 4.21.

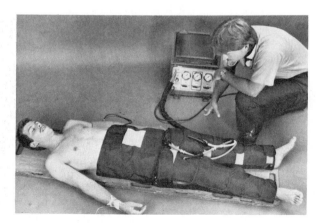

Figure 4.22.

STUDENT NAME _____ **DATE** _____

DIRECTIONS

Evaluate the student by using the criteria presented on this form. Mark PASS for an appropriate action. Mark FAIL for an inappropriate action or missed step. An asterisk (*) indicates an absolute step. Omission of this step indicates automatic failure.

STEP	PASS	FAIL

APPLICATION OF THE ANTI-SHOCK TROUSERS

1. Understands indications* [ ] [ ]
2. Prepares pants on backboard in anticipation of application [ ] [ ]
3. Pulls pants under patient [ ] [ ]
4. Centers patient [ ] [ ]
5. Snugly wraps the legs and seals Velcro fasteners* [ ] [ ]
6. Snugly closes the abdominal compartment [ ] [ ]
7. Connects the inflation tubes [ ] [ ]
8. Closes abdominal valve and inflates the legs first* [ ] [ ]
9. Inflates legs to the proper inflation depending on the brand of trousers being used [ ] [ ]
10. Opens the abdominal valve and inflates the abdominal compartment* [ ] [ ]
11. Checks the vital signs* [ ] [ ]
12. Checks the pedal pulses* [ ] [ ]

REMOVAL OF THE ANTI-SHOCK TROUSERS

13. Understands indications for removal* [ ] [ ]
14. Monitors blood pressure with cuff in place* [ ] [ ]
15. Slowly releases pressure in the abdominal compartment* [ ] [ ]
16. Releases pressure in one leg after complete release of abdominal pressure* [ ] [ ]
17. Releases pressure in the remaining leg compartment after complete release of opposite leg pressure* [ ] [ ]
18. Monitors patient throughout* [ ] [ ]
19. Leaves trousers in place* [ ] [ ]
20. Reevaluates patient [ ] [ ]

TOTAL SCORE (2 points for each PASS) _____
(28 required for PASS)
NO ABSOLUTES MAY BE FAILED

Evaluator _____ Date _____

Application of the Mechanical CPR Device

Overview

The mechanical CPR device is becoming increasingly popular in both pre-hospital and inhospital care. It is designed to mechanically maintain adequate CPR, thus reducing the number of emergency personnel required to manage a cardiac arrest victim.

It offers several advantages over manual CPR. First, it frees emergency personnel to perform advanced life support skills such as defibrillation and medication administration. Second, it reduces the number of personnel required to treat the patient, thus allowing for more room and less confusion. Third, the device is not subject to fatigue and maintains constant CPR as long as appropriately placed. Finally, it can be powered with a portable oxygen source. Thus interruptions in CPR as the patient is moved to or from the ambulance are prevented. However, the device is only for use by qualified personnel and may not be applicable to all situations. Two personnel must be available to properly apply the device.

Indications

Cardiac arrest following the application of standard manual CPR.

Contraindications

The mechanical CPR device generally can be used in any situation where standard manual CPR is indicated. However, EMS personnel should follow local protocols concerning use of the device.

Precautions

The position of the compressor must be monitored constantly, especially after moving the patient. During prolonged transports, it may be necessary to readjust the compression depth.

The mechanical CPR device will quickly deplete portable oxygen sources. Thus, it is important to move the patient as quickly as possible to an oxygen source such as that in the ambulance.

This device is best applied while the patient is on a stretcher or backboard. Also, it is often extremely difficult to move the patient through narrow spaces, such as doorways, with the device in place. When approaching the patient, you should note any obstacles that may make removal of the patient difficult when the device is applied.

Complications

The complications associated with use of the mechanical CPR device are basically the same as those associated with manual CPR. These include fractured ribs and accidental laceration of the heart, lungs, or liver. Because the mechanical CPR device provides automatic ventilation, there is the chance of inadvertently overinflating the lungs which may result in spontaneous pneumothorax.

Required Equipment

- Mechanical CPR device (Figure 4.23)

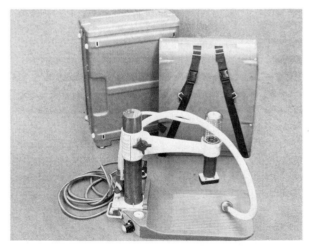

Figure 4.23. The mechanical CPR device.

- Portable oxygen source
- Airway device (mask, ET tube, and/or oral airway)
- Associated tubing
- Required adapters

Procedure

Initiate manual CPR as soon as possible (Figure 4.24).

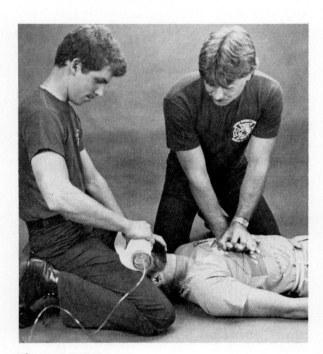

Figure 4.24.

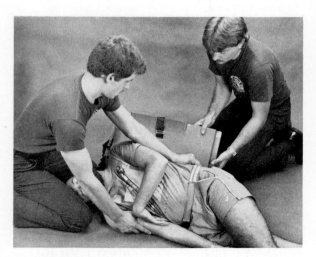

Figure 4.25.

As soon as practical, stop manual CPR, and quickly slide the backboard under the patient (Figure 4.25). Resume CPR.

While maintaining CPR, insert the base plate of the mechanical CPR device into the backboard (Figure 4.26).

Holding the column as shown (Figure 4.27), with the on–off valve toward you, loosen the arm-locking knob, and swing the arm on the column toward the patient's feet. Tighten the arm-locking knob.

Tip the column forward, and slide it into the base (Figure 4.28).

Connect the oxygen input hose (Figure 4.29).

Turn on the master valve and the on–off valve (Figure 4.30).

Verify that the force control knob is turned fully counterclockwise and the ventilator switch is off (Figure 4.31).

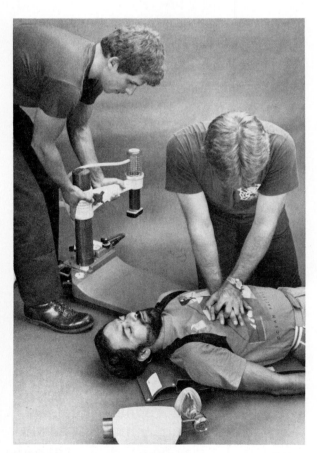

Figure 4.26.

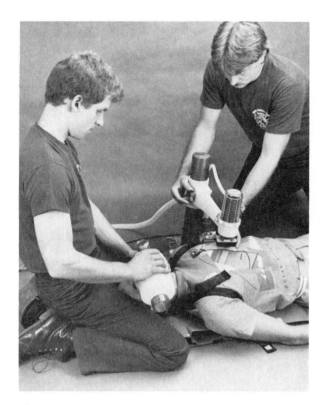

Figure 4.27.

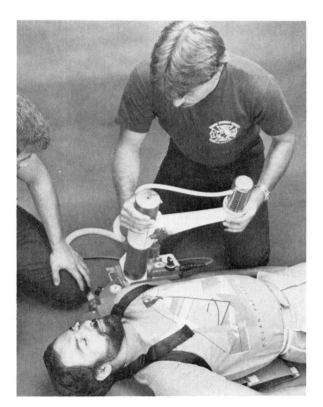

Figure 4.28.

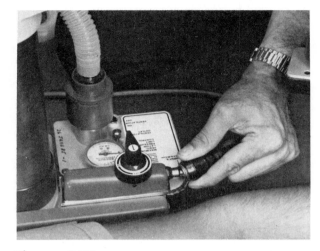

Figure 4.29.

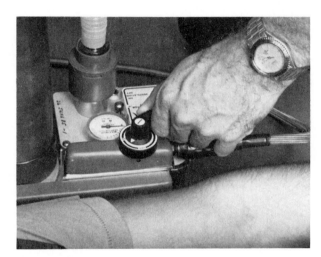

Figure 4.30.

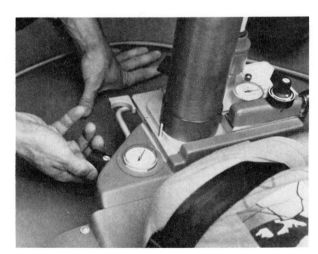

Figure 4.31.

Grab the piston, and raise it into the housing (Figure 4.32). Loosen the arm-locking knob, and swing the arm into the proper position over the patient's sternum.

During the next manual ventilation, quickly position the piston's massager pad on the lower half of the sternum (excluding the xiphoid) (Figure 4.33).

Verify that the bottom white line is just entering the piston housing (Figure 4.34).

Lock the arm in place (Figure 4.35).

Observe the first color piston drawing (Figure 4.36).

Carefully adjust the force-control knob until it matches with the highest visible color line on the mini-color piston drawing (Figure 4.37).

Turn on the ventilator switch, and apply it to the mask, EOA, or ET tube (Figure 4.38).

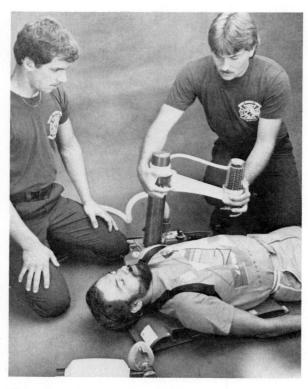

Figure 4.33.

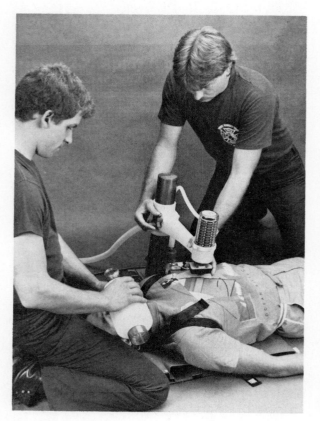

Figure 4.32.

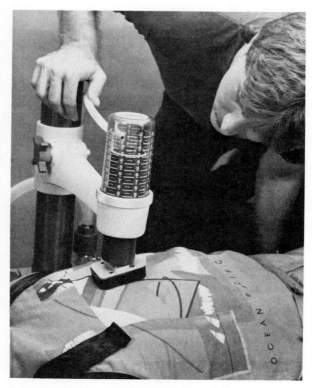

Figure 4.34.

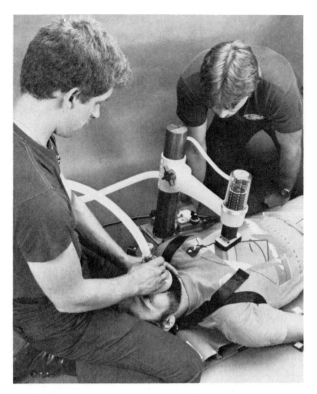

Figure 4.35.

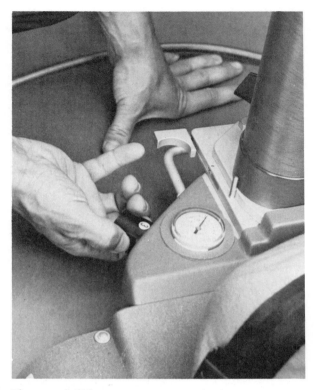

Figure 4.37.

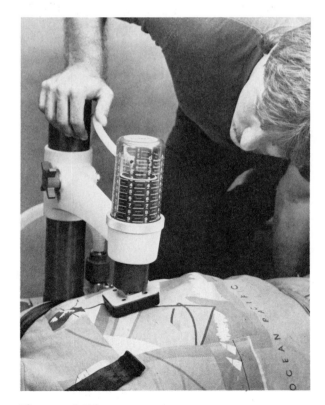

Figure 4.36.

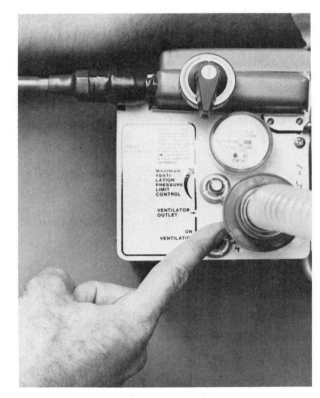

Figure 4.38.

Set the ventilation-control knob to the desired setting (Figure 4.39).

Palpate the femoral and carotid pulses to check the efficiency of the device (Figure 4.40).

Initiate advanced life support procedures (Figure 4.41).

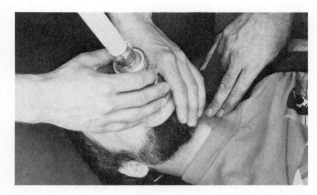

Figure 4.40.

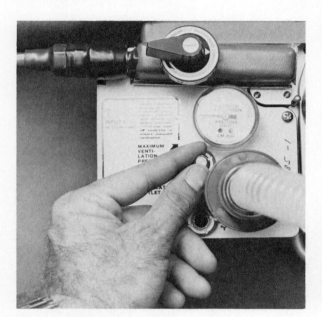

Figure 4.39.

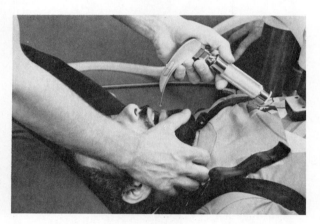

Figure 4.41.

STUDENT NAME ——————————————————— **DATE** ——————————

DIRECTIONS

 Evaluate the student by using the criteria presented on this form. Mark PASS for an appropriate action. Mark FAIL for an inappropriate action or missed step. An asterisk (*) indicates an absolute step. Omission of this step indicates automatic failure.

STEP	PASS	FAIL
APPLICATION OF MECHANICAL CPR DEVICE		
1. Understands indications*	[ ]	[ ]
2. Has partner initiate and maintain manual CPR*	[ ]	[ ]
3. Quickly places backboard under the patient	[ ]	[ ]
4. Inserts base plate into the backboard	[ ]	[ ]
5. Adjusts column out of the way by loosening the arm-lock knob	[ ]	[ ]
6. Slides column into the base	[ ]	[ ]
7. Connects the oxygen input hose	[ ]	[ ]
8. Turns master valve and on–off valve off*	[ ]	[ ]
9. Raises piston into the housing and positions the arm above the patient's sternum in the proper position*	[ ]	[ ]
10. During the next ventilation quickly positions the plunger on the lower half of the sternum (Excluding Xiphoid)*	[ ]	[ ]
11. Verifies white line is just entering the piston housing	[ ]	[ ]
12. Locks the arm in place	[ ]	[ ]
13. Checks color piston drawing	[ ]	[ ]
14. Adjusts force-control knob so that it matches the highest visible color line in the miniature drawing	[ ]	[ ]
15. Turns on ventilator switch	[ ]	[ ]
16. Sets ventilation-control knob to the desired setting	[ ]	[ ]
17. Checks femoral pulses	[ ]	[ ]
18. Reassesses device*	[ ]	[ ]

TOTAL SCORE (2 points for each PASS)   ————————
(25 required for PASS)
NO ABSOLUTES MAY BE FAILED

———————————————————   ———————————————
Evaluator   Date

Insertion of an Indwelling Intravenous Catheter

Overview

The placement of an indwelling intravenous catheter is a fundamental paramedic skill. The procedure involves placing a cannula into either a peripheral or central vein through which various fluids are administered. Generally, in the prehospital setting, IV infusions are of two general types. Trauma IVs are designed for the rapid replacement of fluids that have been lost from the circulatory system for one reason or another. Medical IVs, on the other hand, are designed to maintain direct access to the circulatory system for the administration of medications. Table 4.1 compares trauma and medical IV systems.

Table 4.1.   A Comparison of Trauma and Medical IV Systems.

Feature	Trauma IV	Medical IV
Fluid	lactated Ringer's	5% dextrose
Quantity	1000 mL	500 mL
Administration set	standard set (10–15 gtts/mL)	minidrip set (60 gtts/mL)
Catheter size	14 or 16 gauge	18 or 20 gauge
Infusion rate	fast	slow

Several types of fluids are available for use in prehospital care. However, intravenous fluids can be divided into two general categories, colloids and crystalloids. Colloids contain compounds of high molecular weight, usually proteins, that tend to remain in the circulatory system. Crystalloids, on the other hand, contain only electrolytes and water and tend to diffuse out of the circulatory system. Crystalloids are the most frequently used in prehospital care. Table 4.2. illustrates the various types of crystalloid solutions.

Indications

TRAUMA IV   To replace lost fluids, electrolytes, or blood products.

MEDICAL IV   To maintain immediate access to the circulatory system for the administration of medications.

Contraindications

Intravenous fluids, except as a route for medication administration (TKO), are not indicated in the patient with circulatory overload presenting as either congestive heart failure, pulmonary edema, or a combination of both.

Intravenous fluids may be contraindicated in the chronic dialysis patient. These patients typically have an arteriovenous (AV) shunt in one forearm. If an IV is to be started in these patients it is essential that it be placed in the arm opposite the side of the AV shunt.

Precautions

The blood pressure and the breath sounds must be monitored constantly to prevent circulatory overload. An increase in blood pressure above the desired range or the presence of rales may

Table 4.2. Approximate Ionic Concentrations (mEqL) and Calories per Liter

Solution	Ionic Concentrations (mEq/L)					Calories per liter	Osmolarity[a] (mOsm/L)	pH Range[b]
	Sodium	Potassium	Calcium	Chloride	Lactate			
5% Dextrose Injection, USP	0	0	0	0	0	170	252	3.5–6.5
10% Dextrose Injection, USP	0	0	0	0	0	340	505	3.5–6.5
0.9% Sodium Chloride Injection, USP	154	0	0	154	0	0	308	4.5–7.0
Sodium Lactate Injection, USP (M/6 Sodium Lactate)	167	0	0	0	167	54	334	6.0–7.3
2.5% Dextrose & 0.45% Sodium Chloride Injection, USP	77	0	0	77	0	85	280	3.5–6.0
5% Dextrose & 0.2% Sodium Chloride Injection, USP	34	0	0	34	0	170	321	3.5–6.0
5% Dextrose & 0.33% Sodium Chloride Injection, USP	56	0	0	56	0	170	365	3.5–6.0
5% Dextrose & 0.45% Sodium Chloride Injection, USP	77	0	0	77	0	170	406	3.5–6.0
5% Dextrose & 0.9% Sodium Chloride Injection, USP	154	0	0	154	0	170	560	3.5–6.0
10% Dextrose & 0.9% Sodium Chloride Injection, USP	154	0	0	154	0	340	813	3.5–6.0
Ringer's Injection, USP	147.5	4	4.5	156	0	0	309	5.0–7.5
Lactated Ringer's Injection, USP	130	4	3	109	28	9	273	6.0–7.5
5% Dextrose in Ringer's Injection	147.5	4	4.5	156	0	170	561	3.5–6.5
Lactated Ringer's with 5% Dextrose	130	4	3	109	28	180	525	4.0–6.5

[a] Normal physiolic isotonicity range is approximately 280-310 mOsm/L. Administration of substantially hypotonic solutions may cause hemolysis and administration of substantially hypertonic solutions may cause vein damage.

[b] pH ranges are USP for applicable solution, corporate specification for non-USP solutions.

(From B. Bledsoe, G. Bosker, and F. Papa, *Prehospital Emergency Pharmacology*. Bowie, MD: Brady Communications Company, 1984. Adapted from Travenol Laboratories, Inc., Deerfield, Illinois.)

indicate the early stages of circulatory overload. If these symptoms occur, the flow rate should be cut back significantly or stopped.

Complications

There are many possible complications of IV therapy. A partial list follows.

LOCAL COMPLICATIONS

1. PAIN at the puncture site which may be due to the catheter itself or from extravasation

2. HEMATOMA resulting from the loss of blood into the tissues surrounding the vein

3. INFILTRATION of fluid into the tissue surrounding the vein

4. LOCAL INFECTION due to the introduction of bacteria into the puncture site

5. TISSUE SLOUGHING which occurs from the extravasation of certain drugs or hypertonic solutions (for example, 50% dextrose in water)

SYSTEMIC COMPLICATIONS

1. SYNCOPE occurs quite often and is generally a vasovagal response.

2. SEPSIS can occur from the introduction of bacteria into the circulatory system.

3. AIR EMBOLISM can occur if air is inadvertently allowed to enter the vein. This is especially true in large veins such as the subclavian or the jugular vein.

4. ANAPHYLAXIS can occur following the administration of drugs to which the patient is hypersensitive. Anaphylactic reactions to crystalloids are relatively uncommon.

5. PULMONARY EDEMA can result from fluid overload.

6. PULMONARY THROMBOEM-BOLISM can occur if IV infusions

are left in peripheral leg veins for an extended period of time.

7. CATHETER EMBOLISM can occur if the plastic catheter is sheared off and allowed to enter the circulatory system. To prevent this, the stylet MUST NEVER BE REINSERTED into the cannula once it is removed. It is important to use radiopaque catheters so that the catheter can be located by x ray if it should be inadvertently sheared.

Required Equipment

APPROPRIATE IV FLUID—The type of IV fluid to be administered will depend upon the condition being treated and the personal preference of the base-station physician. Trauma IVs are generally lactated Ringer's or 0.9% sodium chloride. Medical IVs are generally 5% dextrose in water or similar combinations such as 5% dextrose in 0.45% sodium chloride. IV fluids supplied in plastic bags are preferred to those supplied in glass bottles. Do not attempt to mark plastic bags with felt tip markers as the ink may diffuse through both layers of the plastic and contaminate the solution.

ADMINISTRATION SETS—Three types of administration sets are used in pre-hospital care (Figure 4.42): the standard set, the minidrip set, and the Volutrol® or Buretrol® set. A standard set is used with trauma IVs and delivers a much greater quantity of fluid than the other sets (Figure 4.43). A standard set generally delivers 10 drops/mL.

Minidrip sets, on the other hand, deliver fluids much slower and are, thus, easier to calibrate (See Figure 4.43). Most minidrip administration sets deliver 60 drops/mL.

Occasionally, a physician may order the use of the Volutrol or Buretrol administration set. This set is designed for the addition of medications. The medi-

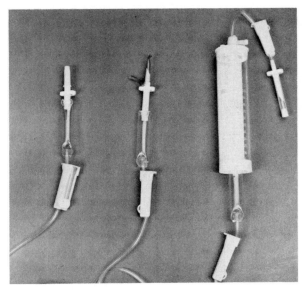

Figure 4.42. Various types of administration sets. Standard set (left), minidrip set (center), and Buretrol set (right).

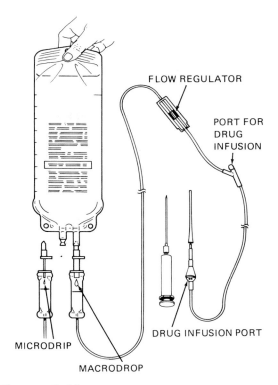

Figure 4.44.

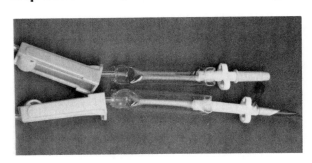

Figure 4.43. Closeup comparing standard and minidrip drip chambers.

cation most commonly delivered via this method is aminophylline. A Buretrol set consists of a medication chamber that hangs below the IV bag itself. A set quantity of fluid can be placed in the medication bag from the IV bag. Medication can then be added to this bag to achieve the proper dilution. Attached to the medication bag is a standard minidrip chamber.

Parts of the IV set are shown in Figure 4.44.

INDWELLING CATHETERS—Several different types of catheters are used in prehospital care. The most common is the catheter over needle type (for example, Angiocath, Quickcath, Medi-cut). With this type of catheter, the catheter and needle are inserted into the vein (Figure 4.45). After the catheter and nee-

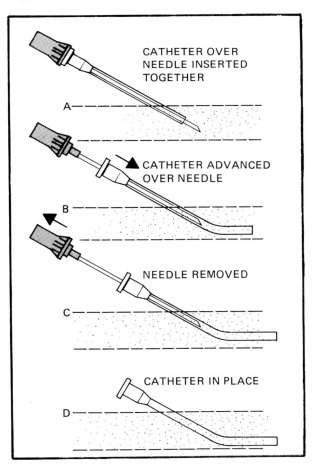

Figure 4.45. Insertion of catheter over needle type of indwelling cannula.

dle have been successfully placed in the vein, the needle is removed and the catheter is left in place.

The catheter through needle (Intracath) is rarely used in prehospital care (Figure 4.46). However, when used, it offers some advantages over the standard catheter over needle device. Catheter through needle devices offer stability and also can provide access to the central circulation. However, Catheter through needle devices are more difficult to insert and have a higher incidence of complications.

The third type of cannula used in prehospital care is the standard winged needle or butterfly catheter (Figure 4.47). This type of catheter is simply inserted into the vein and attached to the

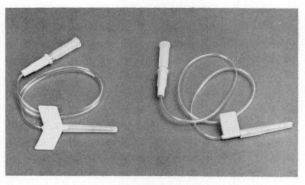

Figure 4.47. Butterfly type cannula.

IV line. It is easy to insert and is often effective when attempting to cannulate extremely small veins or in pediatric cases. Butterfly-type cannulas are not for use in cases where rapid fluid replacement is indicated.

VENOUS CONSTRICTING BAND—A good venous constricting band is essential. These can either be special Velcro tourniquets or simply Penrose drains.

- Extension set
- Antibiotic swabs
- Antiobiotic ointment
- 2×2 Gauze pad
- 1-inch Tape
- Short arm board

Peripheral IV Insertion

The peripheral veins of the forearm, the leg, and occasionally the external jugular vein, are all possible sites for insertion of indwelling catheters. The peripheral veins of the forearm (Figure 4.48) or hand (Figure 4.49) are preferred.

Occasionally, when a vein cannot be located in the forearm, for one reason or another, then the cannula may be placed in a peripheral leg vein (Figure 4.50) or in the external jugular vein (Figure 4.51).

IVs inserted into the peripheral veins of the leg, especially if allowed to remain in place over 24 hours, often lead to phlebitis and possible venous thrombosis. IVs placed in the external jugular vein often are difficult to secure and oc-

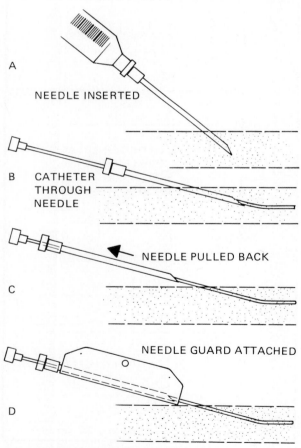

A
NEEDLE INSERTED

B CATHETER THROUGH NEEDLE

NEEDLE PULLED BACK

C

NEEDLE GUARD ATTACHED

D

Figure 4.46. Insertion of a catheter through needle (Intracath) device.

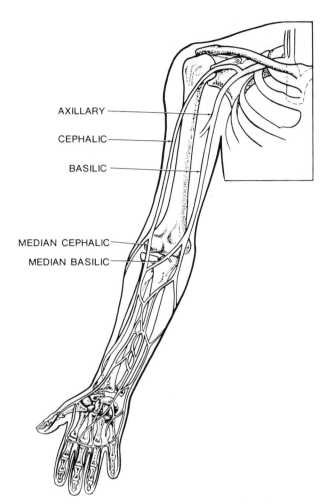

AXILLARY

CEPHALIC

BASILIC

MEDIAN CEPHALIC

MEDIAN BASILIC

Figure 4.48. Peripheral veins of the arm and forearm.

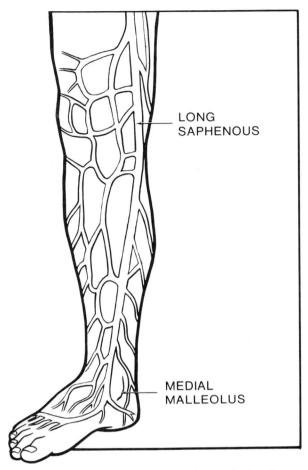

LONG SAPHENOUS

MEDIAL MALLEOLUS

Figure 4.50. Peripheral veins of the leg and thigh.

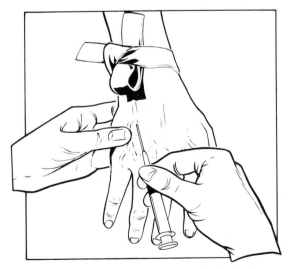

Figure 4.49. Veins of the back of the hand.

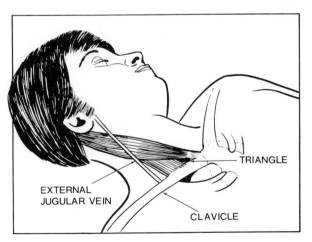

TRIANGLE

EXTERNAL JUGULAR VEIN

CLAVICLE

Figure 4.51. Anatomy of the external jugular vein.

casionally interfere with other medical procedures such as placement of a cervical collar, endotracheal intubation, or general movement of the patient. However, there will be cases where use of these veins may be required and they should be kept in mind.

Procedure

PREPARING THE IV

Select a fluid and inspect for discoloration or the presence of particles in the solution (Figure 4.52). It is common for a little moisture to be present in the packaging envelope.

Locate the notch and tear open the envelope to remove the bag (Figure 4.53).

Again, inspect the fluid for cloudiness or particles. Squeeze the bag to test for possible leaks (Figure 4.54).

Select and open the appropriate administration set (Figure 4.55).

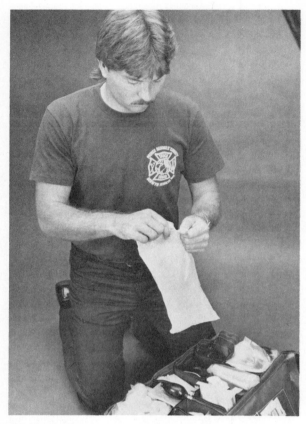

Figure 4.53.

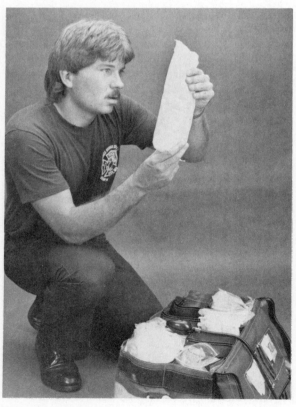

Figure 4.52.

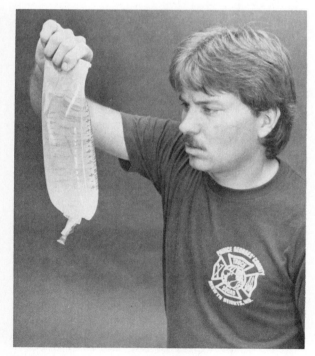

Figure 4.54.

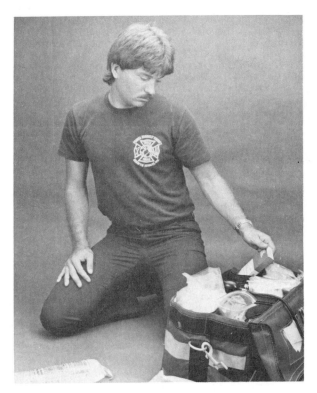

Figure 4.55.

Unroll the administration-set tubing and make sure the control valve is just below the drip chamber (Figure 4.56).

Close the control valve (Figure 4.57).

Remove the protective cap from the distal end of the tubing and connect the extension tube to the administration set (Figure 4.58).

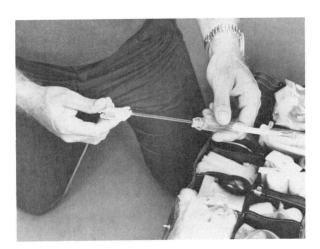

Figure 4.56.

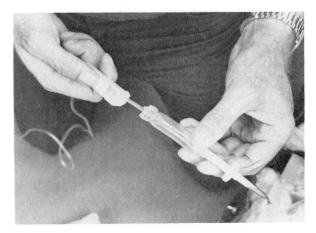

Figure 4.57.

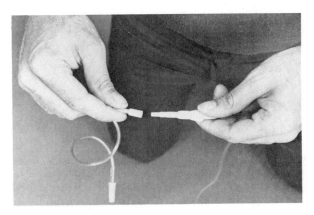

Figure 4.58.

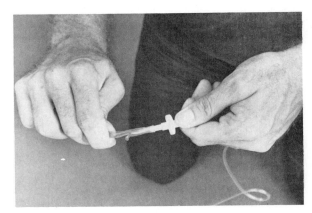

Figure 4.59.

Remove the protective cover from the piercing pin on the administration set and from the port on the IV bag (Figure 4.59).

Insert the piercing pin into the IV bag with a twisting motion (Figure 4.60).

Squeeze the drip chamber and fill it halfway (Figure 4.61).

Uncap the extension tubing (Figure 4.62).

Open the control valve and bleed the air from the line (Figure 4.63).

Close the valve and inspect for the presence of air bubbles in the line (Figure 4.64). If air bubbles are present, bleed the line until they are gone.

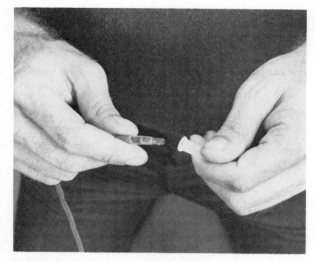

Figure 4.62.

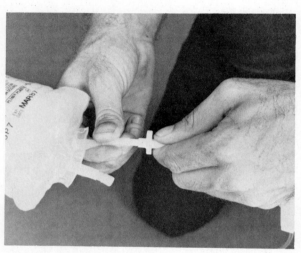

Figure 4.60.

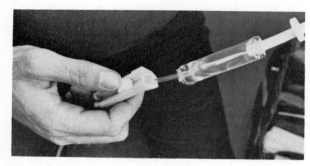

Figure 4.63.

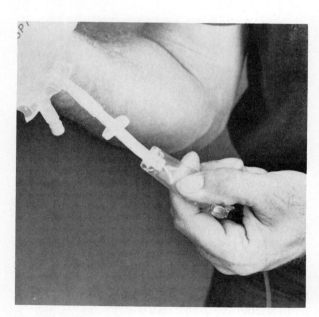

Figure 4.61.

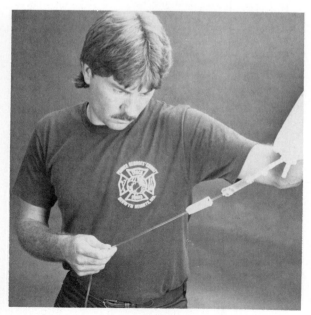

Figure 4.64.

Recap the tubing (Figure 4.65).

Tear off several strips of 1-inch tape and place in a handy location (Figure 4.66). Several commercial IV anchoring devices are available.

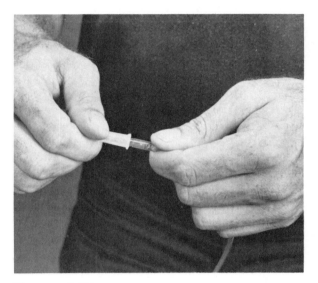

Figure 4.65.

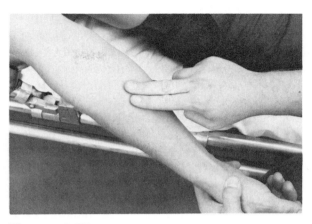

Figure 4.67.

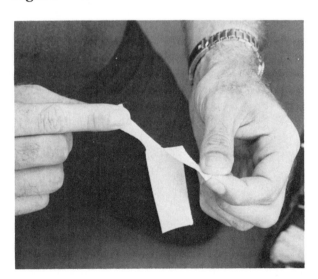

Figure 4.66.

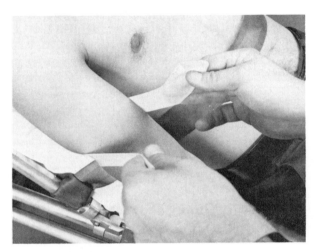

Figure 4.68.

CANNULA INSERTION

Select the arm that appears to have the best veins or is most accessible (Figure 4.67).

Encircle the arm with the venous constricting band (Figure 4.68).

Cross the ends (Figure 4.69).

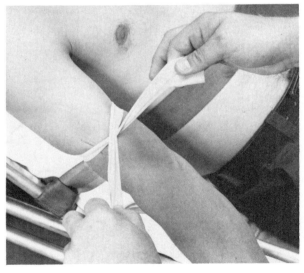

Figure 4.69.

Reach under and tie a slip knot (Figure 4.70). Make sure the ends of the tube do not hang over the proposed puncture site. The constricting band should be applied tight enough to restrict venous flow but not so tight that it affects arterial flow. If in doubt, check the radial pulse.

Palpate a suitable vein (Figure 4.71).

Prep the site with an antiseptic solution (Figure 4.72). Start at the center and work outward with a circular motion.

If desired, remove any providone iodine with an alcohol prep (Figure 4.73).

The needle should be turned so that the bevel is up as you begin to make the puncture (Figure 4.74).

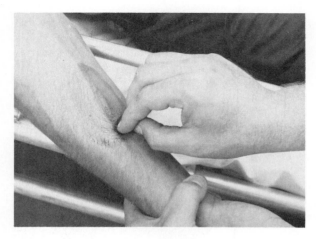

Figure 4.72.

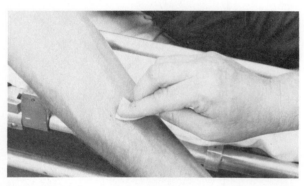

Figure 4.73.

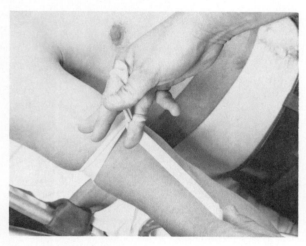

Figure 4.70.

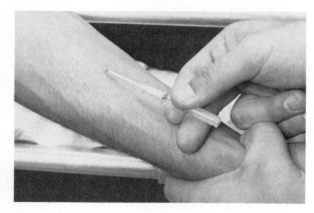

Figure 4.74.

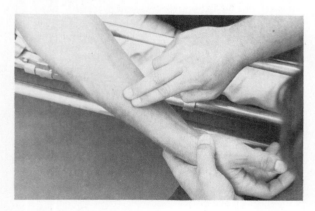

Figure 4.71.

Enter the skin in a steady, deliberate fashion (Figure 4.75).

Continue with the puncture and enter the vein (Figure 4.76). Some resistance will be noted as you puncture the wall of the vein. This will usually be followed by

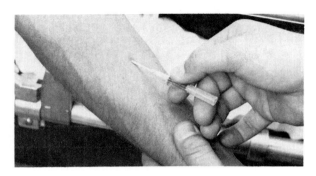

Figure 4.75.

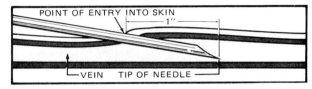

POINT OF ENTRY INTO SKIN
1"
VEIN   TIP OF NEEDLE

Figure 4.76.

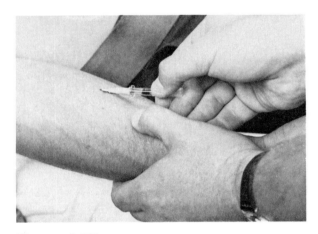

Figure 4.77.

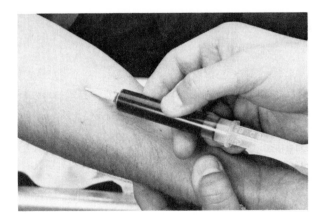

Figure 4.78.

a blood return as you enter the lumen of the vein.

After blood return is noted, advance the catheter into the vein while holding the needle constant (Figure 4.77).

If required, take a blood sample (Figure 4.78).

Apply pressure above the site of the puncture to reduce or stop blood flow as you connect the IV tubing (Figure 4.79).

Remove the constricting band (Figure 4.80).

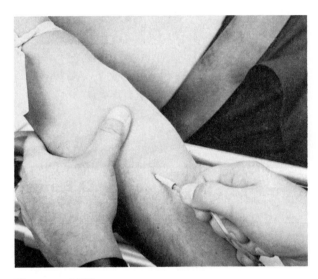

Figure 4.79.

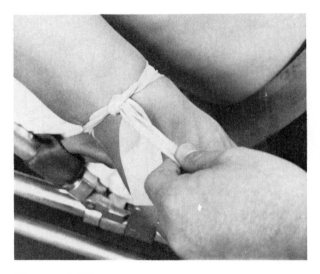

Figure 4.80.

Open the control valve and note the quality of flow (Figure 4.81).

Inspect the tissue around the puncture site for infiltration (Figure 4.82). If noted, discontinue the IV infusion at once.

Apply an antibacterial ointment to the puncture site (Figure 4.83).

Place a 2×2 gauze pad over the puncture site (Figure 4.84).

Place a piece of tape around the catheter in the manner shown or as directed by your medical director or training institution (Figure 4.85).

Complete taping (Figure 4.86).

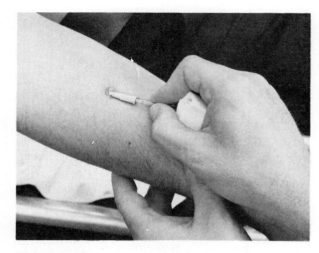

Figure 4.83.

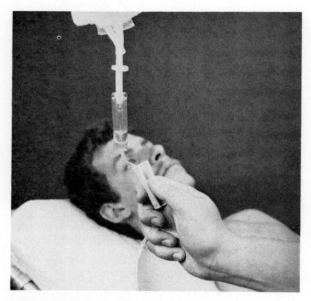

Figure 4.81.

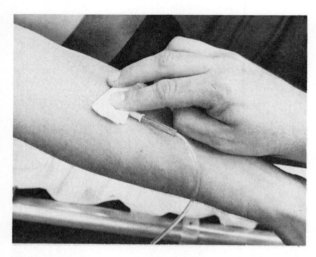

Figure 4.84.

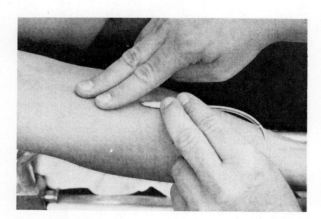

Figure 4.82.

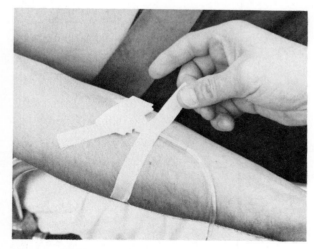

Figure 4.85.

Make any required adjustments to the flow rate (Figure 4.87).

Label the puncture site with the type and gauge of catheter, the time the IV was started, and your initials (Figure 4.88).

If necessary, stabilize the arm with a short arm board (figure 4.89).

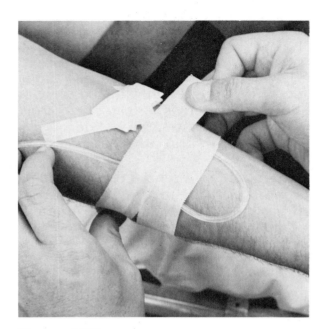

Figure 4.86.

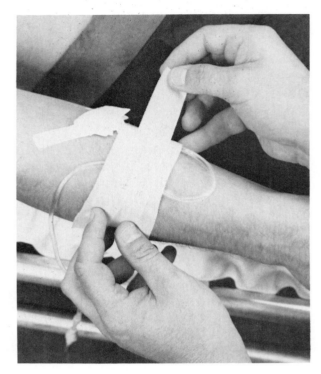

Figure 4.88.

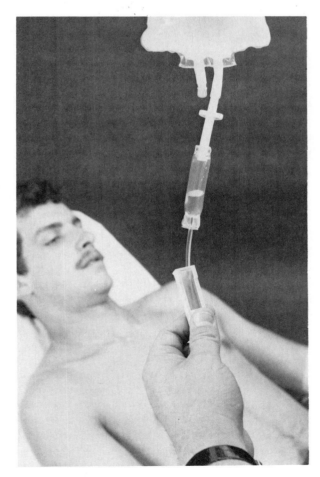

Figure 4.87.

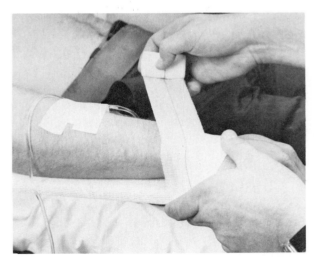

Figure 4.89.

TROUBLESHOOTING THE IV

Many times an IV will not flow as desired. The following steps should be followed in an attempt to localize and remedy the problem.

1. Make sure the venous constricting band has been removed. Also make sure that the patient is not wearing tight clothing which may restrict venous flow.

2. Check the IV puncture site for swelling or infiltration.

3. Check all tubing valves to assure that they are open. Be sure to check the valve on the extension set.

4. If the drip chamber is completely filled, invert the IV bag and squeeze the drip chamber to allow some of the fluid to return to the bag.

5. If flow is still slow or absent, lower the bag below the level of the insertion site and inspect for free blood return into the IV tubing. This indicates patency of the IV. If problems still persist, discontinue the IV and reattempt in the opposite extremity.

CENTRAL VEIN CANNULATION

The placement of central lines is not a routine prehospital skill. However, it is recognized that several EMS systems exist where paramedics are called upon to place central lines, most often when a peripheral line cannot be placed.

The cannulation of central veins is more complicated and often more difficult than the cannulation of peripheral veins. There are several advantages to central vein cannulation. First, central veins can be cannulated even in the presence of circulatory collapse. Second, they allow a greater rate of fluid administration than peripheral veins.

However, there are also several disadvantages. First, the technique of central venous cannulation requires considerable skill and practice. A functional knowledge of gross anatomy is essential. Second, the insertion of a central line often requires the interruption of CPR. Finally, there is a greater likelihood of causing injury to arteries, nerves, or other nearby structures such as the lungs.

There are three central veins routinely cannulated. These are the internal jugular, the subclavian, and the femoral. A thorough understanding of the gross anatomy of the area surrounding these structures is essential.

Prior to attempting cannulation of the jugular or the subclavian vein, the patient should be placed in a supine, head down (Trendelenberg) of at least 15° to distend the veins and to reduce the chances of air embolism. In addition, the technique should be considered a surgical technique, therefore, sterile gloves are used and appropriate draping is applied.

This text will not present a detailed discussion of these techniques. These procedures can only be learned in the cadaver laboratory or morgue under the instruction of a qualified instructor.

INTERNAL JUGULAR CANNULATION

The internal jugular vein is a large vein that drains the head and neck (Figure 4.90). It passes immediately under the sternocleidomastoid muscle and joins the subclavian vein.

The right internal jugular vein is preferred because: (1) the dome of the pleura of the right lung is lower than in the left, (2) there is a straight line to the right atrium, and (3) the thoracic duct is present on the left.

There are three approaches to the internal jugular vein. The posterior approach involves passing the needle along the posterior border of the sternocleidomastoid muscle (Figure 4.91).

The central approach involves inserting the needle at the triangle between the sternal and clavicular heads of the sternocleidomastoid muscle (Figure 4.92). Finally, the anterior approach involves inserting the needle at the anterior border of the sternocleidomastoid muscle (Figure 4.93).

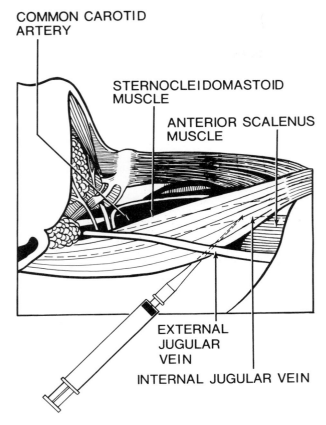

Figure 4.90. Anatomy of the internal jugular vein.

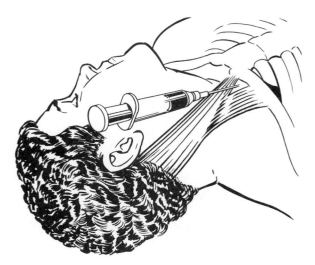

Figure 4.92. Central approach to the cannulation of the internal jugular vein.

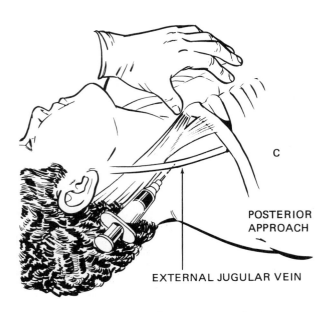

Figure 4.91. Posterior approach to cannulation of the internal jugular vein.

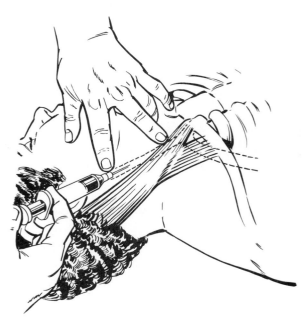

Figure 4.93. Anterior approach to cannulation of the internal jugular vein.

SUBCLAVIAN VEIN CANNULATION

The subclavian vein is a large vein that drains the arm (Figure 4.94). It passes immediately under the clavicle and combines with the internal jugular vein.

Cannulation of the subclavian vein involves inserting a needle around the clavicle and into the vein (Figure 4.95).

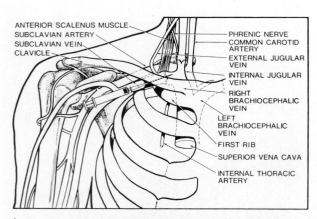

Figure 4.94. Anatomy of the subclavian vein.

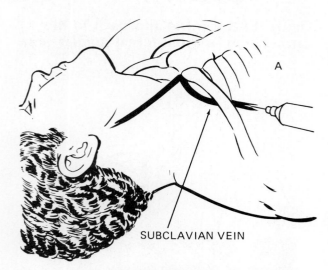

Figure 4.95. Infraclavicular subclavian venipuncture.

FEMORAL VEIN CANNULATION

The femoral vein lies in the femoral sheath and drains the legs (Figure 4.96). The vein lies medial to the femoral artery immediately below the inguinal ligament.

Cannulation of the femoral vein (Figure 4.97) has a slight advantage over internal jugular and subclavian cannulation; CPR does not have to be interrupted for cannulation. In addition, the catheter is often easier to secure than in the other approaches.

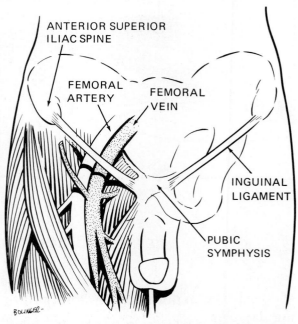

Figure 4.96. Anatomy of the femoral vein.

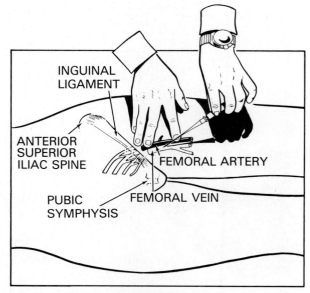

Figure 4.97. Cannulation of the femoral vein.

Discontinuation of IV Therapy

Occasionally the paramedic may be called upon to discontinue an IV in the field. This may be due to either a problem with the IV or refusal of the patient to go to the hospital. The classic case involves the unconscious diabetic patient in hypoglycemia. Paramedics respond and treat the patient appropriately with an IV of 5% dextrose in water and 50 mL of 50% dextrose. After administration of the drug, the patient regains consciousness and refuses to be transported to the hospital. In this case, the paramedics must discontinue the IV.

The primary concern in discontinuing an IV is to avoid inducing infection and catheter embolism.

Reduce the flow rate to "TKO" (Figure 4.98).

Remove all of the tape from the puncture site (Figure 4.99). Do not remove the 2×2 gauze pad and antibacterial ointment covering the puncture site.

Although not generally required, it is a good idea to apply a venous constricting band above the puncture site in much the same manner as was used when making the venipuncture (Figure 4.100). In the event of an inadvertent catheter embolism, the venous constricting band will prevent the catheter from entering the central circulation.

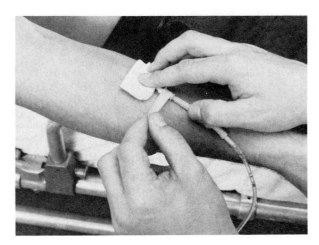

Figure 4.99.

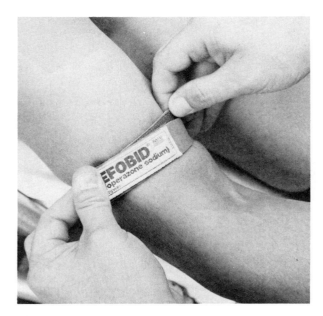

Figure 4.100.

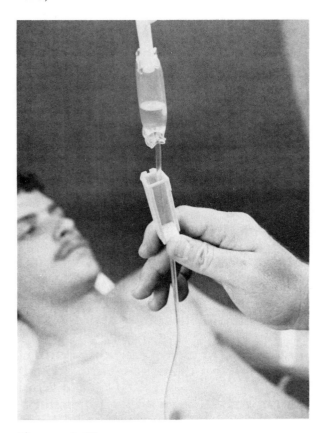

Figure 4.98.

Completely shut the flow valve (Figure 4.101).

With a steady, deliberate action remove the catheter (Figure 4.102).

Maintain pressure on the puncture site with the 2×2 gauze pad already in place (Figure 4.103).

After maintaining pressure for a minute or so, remove the gauze pad and inspect the site (Figure 4.104).

Reapply fresh antibacterial ointment and apply a Band-Aid (Figure 4.105).

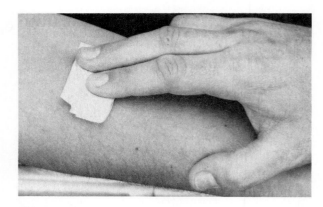

Figure 4.103.

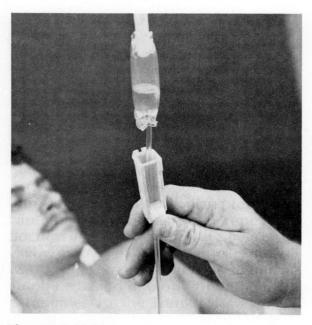

Figure 4.101.

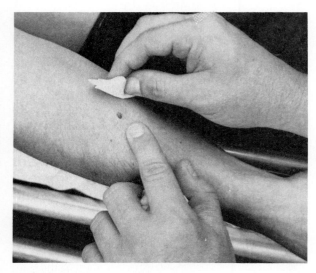

Figure 4.104.

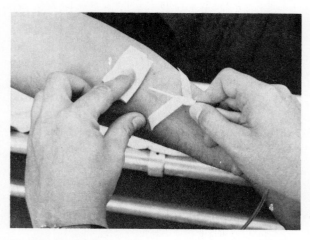

Figure 4.102.

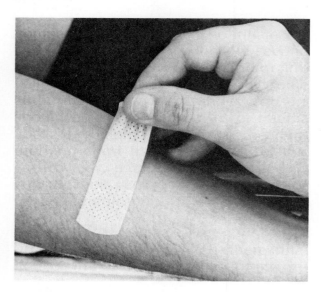

Figure 4.105.

STUDENT NAME _____ **DATE** _____

DIRECTIONS

Evaluate the student by using the criteria presented on this form. Mark PASS for an appropriate action. Mark FAIL for an inappropriate action or missed step. An asterisk (*) indicates an absolute step. Omission of this step indicates automatic failure.

STEP	PASS	FAIL
PREPARATION OF THE IV INFUSION		
1. Receives the order*	[ ]	[ ]
2. Selects proper fluid and inspects for particles or discoloration*	[ ]	[ ]
3. Opens the envelope	[ ]	[ ]
4. Selects the appropriate administration set*	[ ]	[ ]
5. Unrolls tubing and positions the drip rate control valve	[ ]	[ ]
6. Closes the control valve	[ ]	[ ]
7. Connects extension tubing	[ ]	[ ]
8. Removes protective cover and inserts administration set into bag by using aseptic technique*	[ ]	[ ]
9. Squeezes the drip chamber to prime the administration set	[ ]	[ ]
10. Bleeds all of the air from the line	[ ]	[ ]
11. Closes the valve and inspects for air bubbles in the line*	[ ]	[ ]
12. Recaps the tubing*	[ ]	[ ]
CANNULA INSERTION		
13. Selects best arm	[ ]	[ ]
14. Places tourniquet and palpates a suitable vein	[ ]	[ ]
15. Preps the site with an antibacterial swab*	[ ]	[ ]
16. Turns needle so that the bevel is up and punctures the vein	[ ]	[ ]
17. Takes blood sample	[ ]	[ ]
18. Applies pressure above the site of the puncture and connects IV tubing to the cannula	[ ]	[ ]
19. Removes the tourniquet	[ ]	[ ]
20. Opens the control valve and notes the quality of flow*	[ ]	[ ]
21. Inspects the tissue around the puncture site for infiltration*	[ ]	[ ]
22. Applies ointment	[ ]	[ ]
23. Secures catheter and line	[ ]	[ ]
24. Adjusts flow rate as ordered*	[ ]	[ ]
25. Labels bag	[ ]	[ ]
26. Confirms IV placement with the base-station physician	[ ]	[ ]

TOTAL SCORE (2 points for each PASS) _____
(36 required for PASS)
NO ABSOLUTES MAY BE FAILED

_____   _____
Evaluator   Date

Chapter Objectives

Upon completion of this chapter, the student should be able to:

1. List the indications, contraindications, precautions, and common complications of the following procedures:

   a. Subcutaneous injection
   b. Intramuscular injection
   c. Intravenous drug administration (bolus)
   d. Intravenous drug administration (piggyback)
   e. Dextrostix for blood glucose analysis
   f. Transtracheal medication instillation
   g. Intracardiac injection
   h. Nitronox administration
   i. Nasogastric tube insertion

2. Be able to perform the following procedures according to the criteria presented:

   a. Subcutaneous injection
   b. Intramuscular injection
   c. Intravenous drug administration (bolus)
   d. Intravenous drug administration (piggyback)
   e. Dextrostix for blood glucose analysis
   f. Transtracheal medication instillation
   g. Intracardiac injection
   h. Nitronox administration
   i. Nasogastric tube insertion

5

Medication Administration Skills

Subcutaneous Injection

Overview

The subcutaneous route of medication administration is rarely used in prehospital care. With subcutaneous administration, medications are injected into the fatty, subcutaneous tissue under the skin and overlying the muscle. The rate of absorption is slower than that seen with intramuscular and intravenous administration. Epinephrine 1:1000, which is used in the treatment of acute asthma and other similar respiratory emergencies, is almost always administered subcutaneously. A maximum of 2 mL of a drug can be administered subcutaneously.

Indications

Subcutaneous injection is indicated when a relatively slow rate of medication absorption is desired.

Contraindications

Subcutaneous administration is not indicated for patients in shock who often have peripheral vasoconstriction which will slow medication absorption significantly.

Precautions

It is essential to assure that the patient is not allergic to any medications before administering the drug. It is also important to choose a part of the body that has a good pad of subcutaneous tissue and where there are no major arteries, veins, or nerves. The subcutaneous tissue over the deltoid muscle is the most commonly used.

It is important to aspirate the syringe to assure that a blood vessel has not been entered before administering the medication.

Complications

Infection, hematoma, local tissue irritation, and accidental IV administration are all complications of subcutaneous administration. Most of these can be avoided by using proper technique.

Required Equipment

- 1-mL Syringe
- Alcohol prep
- Medication
- Needle (⅝", 25 gauge)
- 4×4 Gauze pad
- Band-Aid

Procedure

Receive the order (Figure 5.1).
Confirm the order and write it down (Figure 5.2).
Prepare the necessary equipment (Figure 5.3).

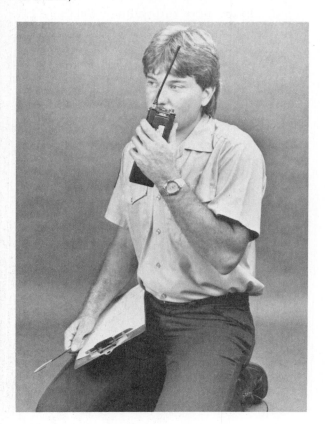

Figure 5.1.

Twist the needle so that it is firmly attached to the syringe (Figure 5.4).

Explain to the patient what you are going to do (Figure 5.5). Reconfirm that the patient is not allergic to any medications.

Select the medication (Figure 5.6).

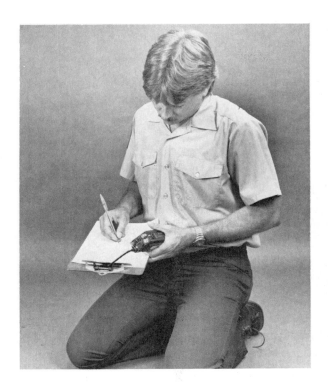

Figure 5.2.

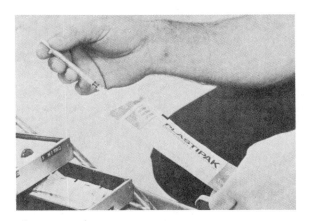

Figure 5.3.

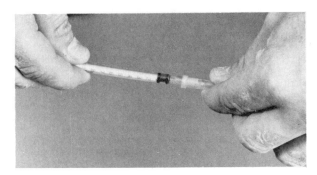

Figure 5.4.

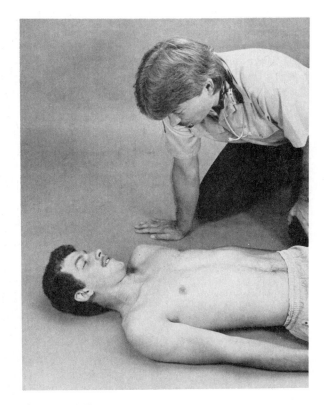

Figure 5.5.

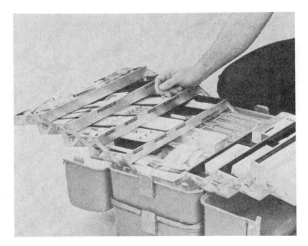

Figure 5.6.

Read the name of the medication and inspect the solution for discoloration or the presence of particles (Figure 5.7).

"Shake down" the ampule to force the liquid to the bottom of the vial so that it can be broken without spillage (Figure 5.8).

Break the ampule by using a 4×4 gauze pad to prevent injury (Figure 5.9).

Insert the needle downward (Figure 5.10).

Withdraw the medication (Figure 5.11).

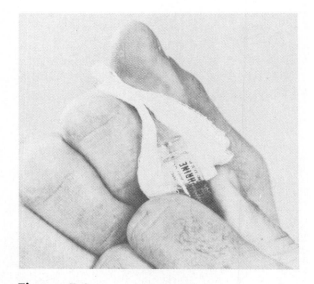

Figure 5.9.

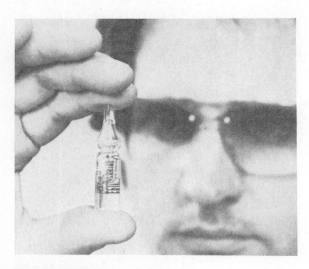

Figure 5.7.

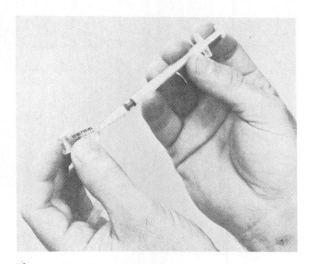

Figure 5.10.

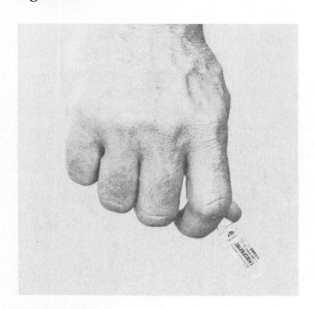

Figure 5.8.

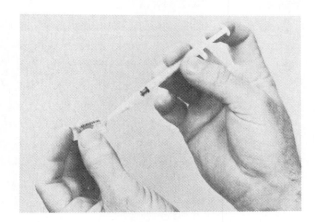

Figure 5.11.

Insert the needle into the inverted ampule (Figure 5.12).

Withdraw the remaining medication (Figure 5.13).

Expel any air present (Figure 5.14).

Recap the needle (Figure 5.15).

Properly dispose of the broken ampule (Figure 5.16).

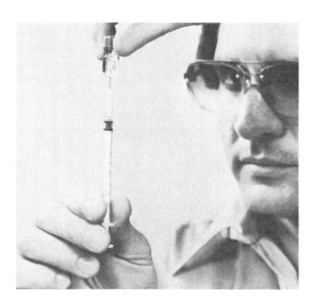

Figure 5.12.

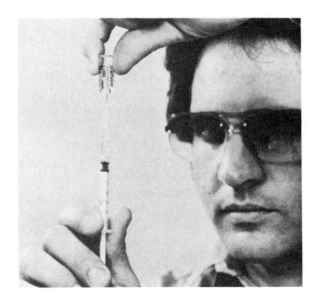

Figure 5.13.

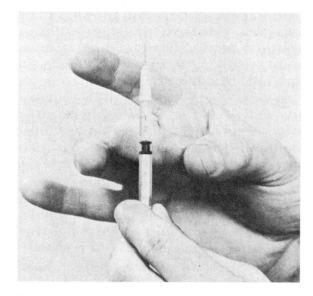

Figure 5.14.

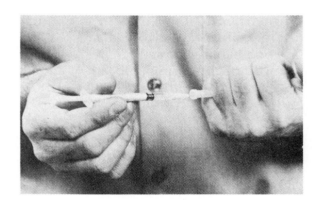

Figure 5.15.

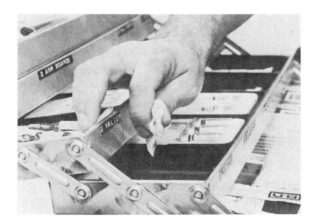

Figure 5.16.

Expose the deltoid (Figure 5.17).
Prep the deltoid with an alcohol swab (Figure 5.18).
Insert the needle at a 45° angle to skin (Figure 5.19).
Needle properly in subcutaneous tissue (Figure 5.20).
Aspirate for blood (Figure 5.21).
Inject the medication (Figure 5.22).
Apply pressure to the site (Figure 5.23).
If necessary, apply a Band-Aid (Figure 5.24).
Properly dispose of the syringe and needle (Figure 5.25).
Confirm administration of the medication (Figure 5.26).

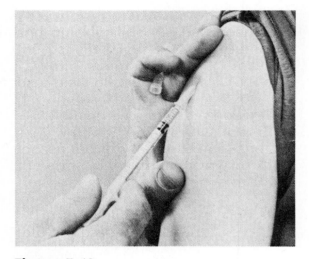
Figure 5.19.

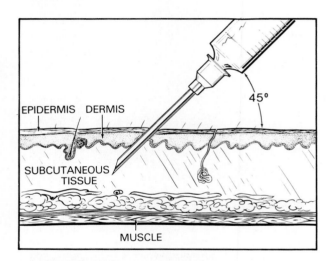
Figure 5.20.

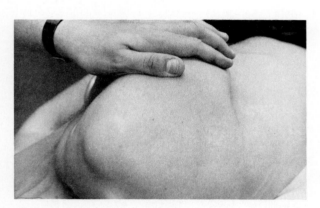
Figure 5.17.

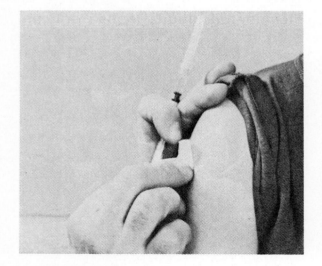
Figure 5.18.

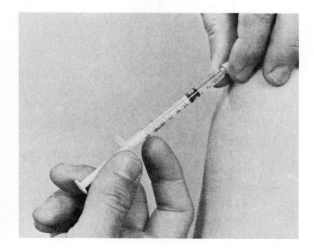
Figure 5.21.

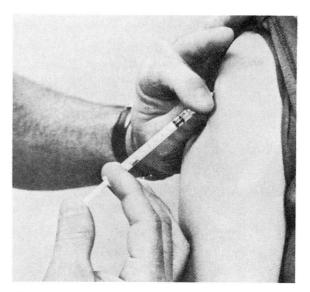

Figure 5.22.

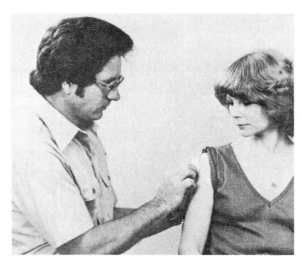

Figure 5.23.

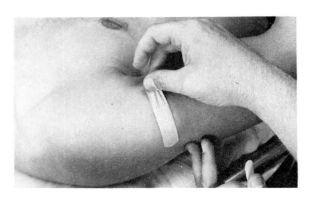

Figure 5.24.

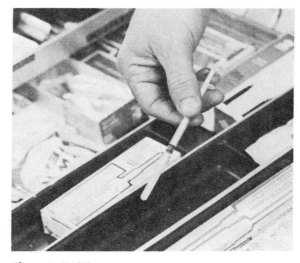

Figure 5.25.

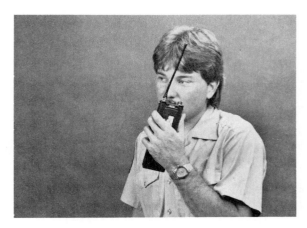

Figure 5.26.

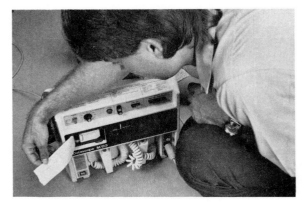

Figure 5.27.

Monitor the patient for the desired therapeutic effects as well as any possible side effects (Figure 5.27).

STUDENT NAME _____ **DATE** _____

DIRECTIONS

Evaluate the student by using the criteria presented on this form. Mark PASS for an appropriate action. Mark FAIL for an inappropriate action or missed step. An asterisk (*) indicates an absolute step. Omission of this step indicates automatic failure.

	STEP	PASS	FAIL
1.	Prepares the necessary equipment	[ ]	[ ]
2.	Explains procedure to the patient	[ ]	[ ]
3.	Reconfirms patient is not allergic to the medication*	[ ]	[ ]
4.	Selects the correct medication*	[ ]	[ ]
5.	Inspects medication for discoloration, particles, and checks expiration date	[ ]	[ ]
6.	"Shakes down" the ampule	[ ]	[ ]
7.	Properly breaks the ampule	[ ]	[ ]
8.	Withdraws medication properly	[ ]	[ ]
9.	Chooses appropriate site*	[ ]	[ ]
10.	Preps site with alcohol prep*	[ ]	[ ]
11.	Inserts needle at 45° angle*	[ ]	[ ]
12.	Aspirates for blood*	[ ]	[ ]
13.	Injects medication*	[ ]	[ ]
14.	Applies pressure to site	[ ]	[ ]
15.	Monitors patient and records administration on chart	[ ]	[ ]

TOTAL SCORE (2 points for each PASS)   _____
(20 required for PASS)
NO ABSOLUTES MAY BE FAILED

_____   _____

Evaluator   Date

Intramuscular Injection
Overview

Intramuscular injection is useful when a relatively rapid drug action is not required or desired. The medication is injected into muscle tissue where it is absorbed into the bloodstream. Absorption is somewhat faster than with subcutaneous injection because muscle tissue is more vascular than subcutaneous tissue. The most common muscles into which drugs are administered are the deltoid and the gluteus. A maximum of 1 mL of medication can be administered into the deltoid while a minimum of 5 mL can be given into the gluteus.

Indications

Intramuscular injection is indicated in non-cardiac emergencies where a relatively slow rate of medication absorption is desired.

Contraindications

Intramuscular injection is not indicated for patients in shock who usually have peripheral vasoconstriction which slows medication absorption significantly. Also, if shock is suddenly reversed, a large quantity of the drug may be absorbed all at once.

Intramuscular (IM) injections should not be given to patients with suspected myocardial infarction. IM injections, since they cause local muscle damage, frequently cause an elevation of circulating muscle enzymes [for example, lactate dehydrogenase (LDH)]. Emergency physicians frequently perform an analysis of these enzymes to detect whether or not cardiac muscle damage has occurred. Thus, IM injections can elevate the enzyme levels and confuse the physician and possibly prevent a speedy diagnosis.

Precautions

It is essential to assure that the patient is not allergic to the medication you are going to administer. You must also choose a proper site and administer the medication properly.

It is important to aspirate the syringe to assure that a blood vessel has not been entered before administering the medication.

Complications

Local pain and burning are common complications associated with IM injection. These complications will vary with the quantity and type of medication administered. Local infection, hematoma, and inadvertent IV injection are also possible.

Required Equipment

- Syringe of sufficient size to contain the medication
- Needle (preferably 1½ inch in length, 21 gauge)
- Alcohol prep
- 4 × 4 Gauze pad
- Medication

Procedure

Receive order and write it down (Figure 5.28).

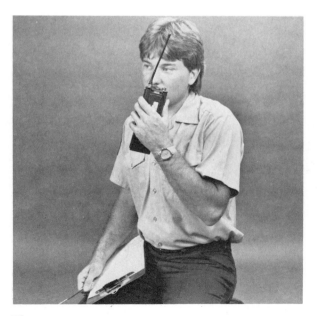

Figure 5.28.

Confirm the order (Figure 5.29).

Prepare the necessary equipment (Figure 5.30).

Twist the needle to confirm that it is firmly attached (Figure 5.31).

Explain to the patient what you are going to do and reconfirm that the patient is not allergic to the medication (Figure 5.32).

Select the medication (Figure 5.33).

Read the name on the medication and inspect the solution for discoloration or the presence of particles (Figure 5.34).

"Shake down" the ampule to force the liquid to the bottom so that it will not spill when broken (Figure 5.35).

Break the ampule by using a 4 × 4 gauze pad to prevent injury (Figure 5.36).

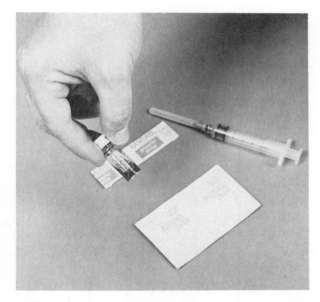

Figure 5.30.

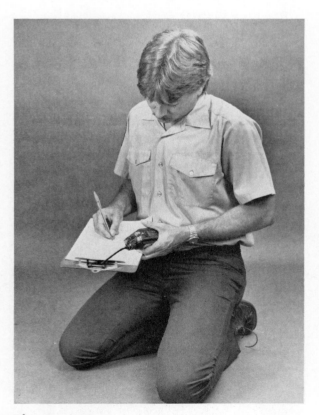

Figure 5.29.

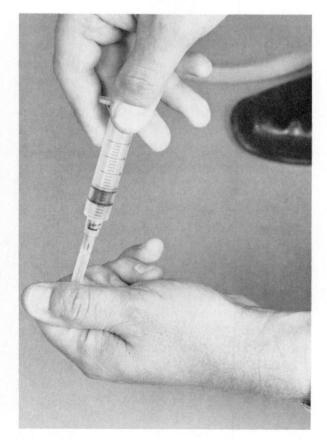

Figure 5.31.

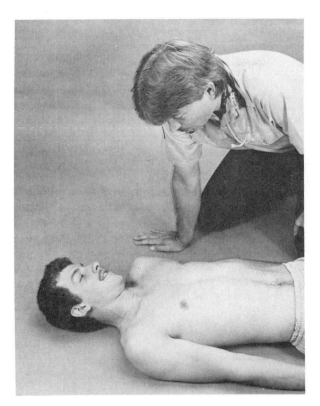

Figure 5.32.

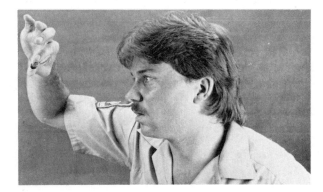

Figure 5.34.

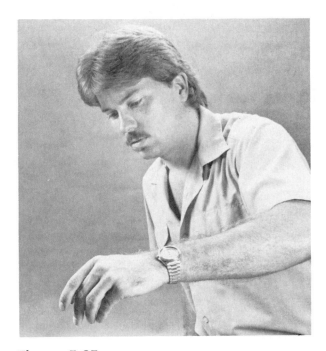

Figure 5.35.

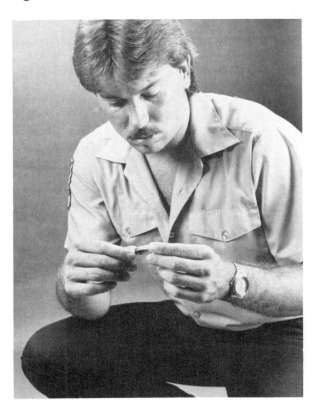

Figure 5.33.

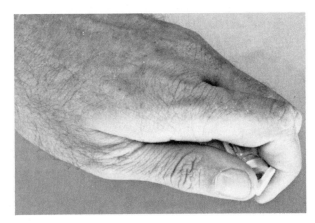

Figure 5.36.

Withdraw the medication (Figure 5.37).

Invert the syringe and expel any air present (Figure 5.38).

Recap the needle (Figure 5.39).

Properly dispose of the ampule (Figure 5.40).

Expose the deltoid or gluteus (Figure 5.41).

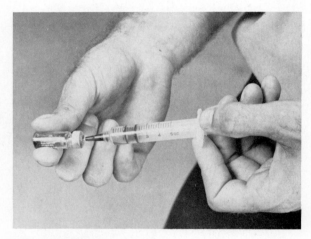

Figure 5.37.

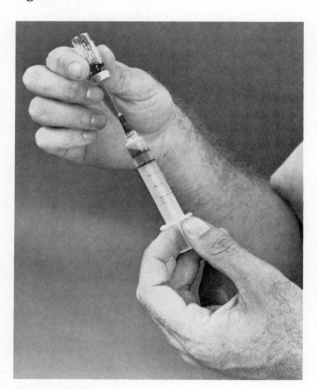

Figure 5.38.

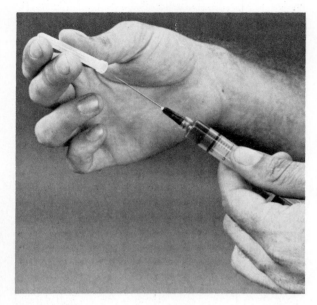

Figure 5.39.

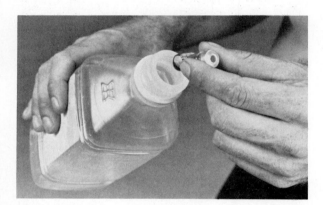

Figure 5.40.

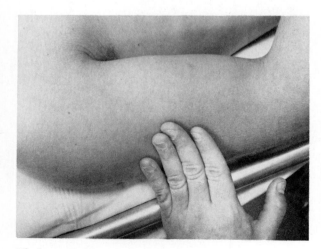

Figure 5.41.

Anatomy of the deltoid region (Figure 5.42).

Anatomy of the gluteal region (Figure 5.43).

Prep the site with an alcohol swab (Figure 5.44).

Insert the needle at a 90° angle (Figure 5.45).

Place needle in proper position for administration (Figure 5.46).

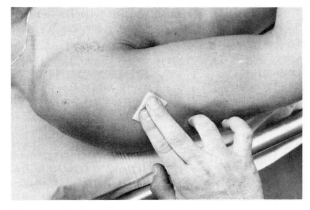

Figure 5.44.

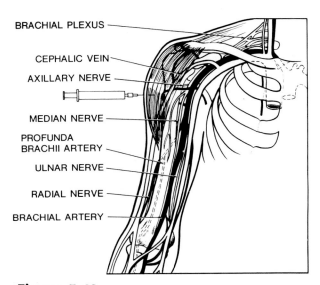

Figure 5.42.

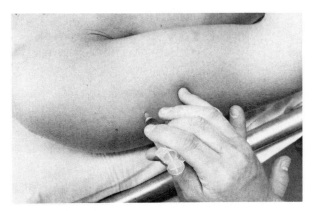

Figure 5.45.

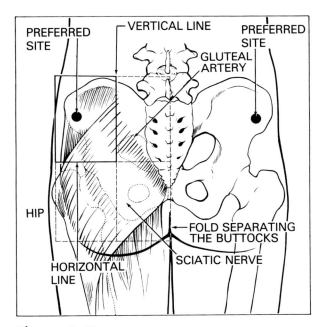

Figure 5.43.

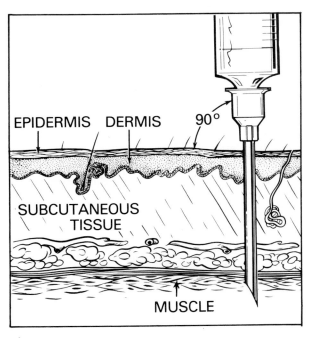

Figure 5.46.

Aspirate to assure that a blood vessel has not been entered (Figure 5.47).

Inject the medication in a slow, deliberate fashion (Figure 5.48).

Apply pressure to the site (Figure 5.49).

If necessary, apply a Band-Aid (Figure 5.50).

Properly dispose of the syringe and needle (Figure 5.51).

Confirm medication administration (Figure 5.52).

Monitor the patient for the desired therapeutic effects as well as any possible side effects (Figure 5.53).

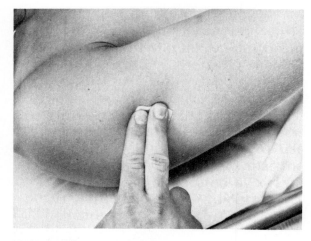

Figure 5.49.

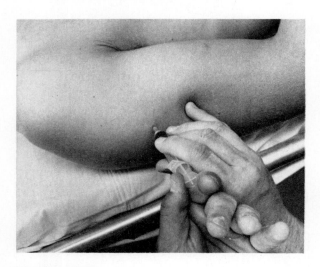

Figure 5.47.

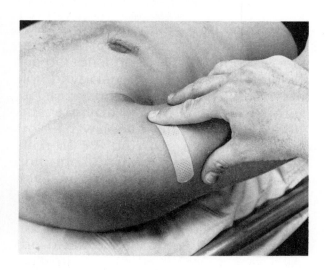

Figure 5.50.

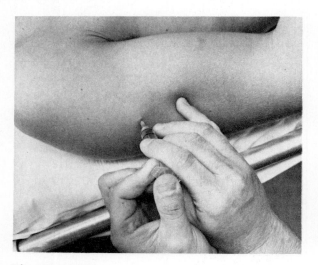

Figure 5.48.

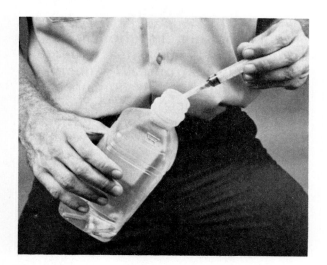

Figure 5.51.

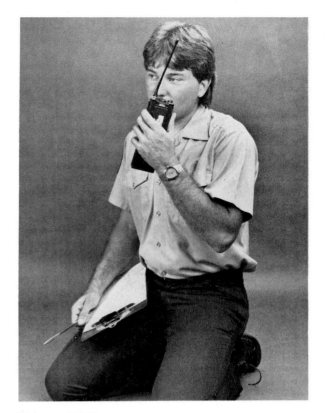

Figure 5.52.

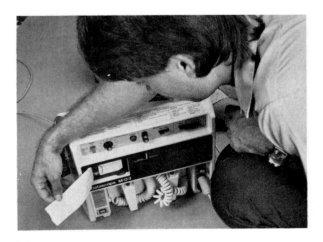

Figure 5.53.

Alternate Injection Technique
"Z-Track"

There is an alternate technique to that described above; it is commonly referred to as "z-track." This technique is preferred by many and is especially useful in thin individuals or when a large quantity of medication is to be injected. Before the skin is punctured, it is slid to one side (Figures 5.54 and 5.55). The injection is made (Figures 5.56 and 5.57),

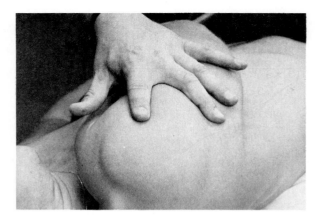

Figure 5.54.

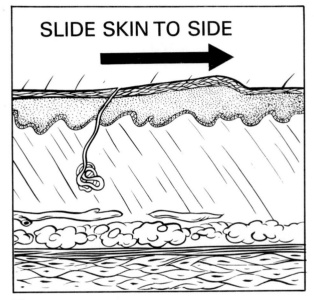

SLIDE SKIN TO SIDE

Figure 5.55.

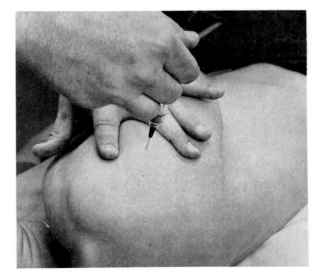

Figure 5.56.

159

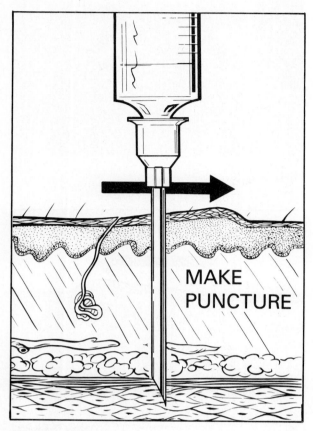

Figure 5.57.

and the skin is allowed to return to its normal position (Figures 5.58 and 5.59) thus effectively sealing the puncture site.

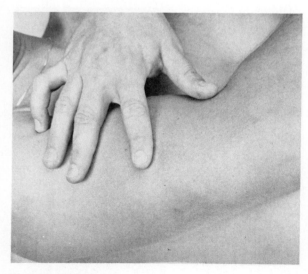

Figure 5.58.

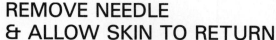
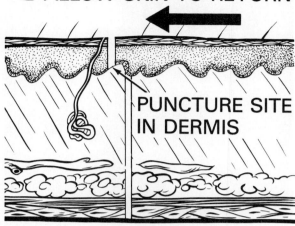

Figure 5.59.

THE TUBEX® SYSTEM

The Tubex system (Wyeth Laboratories) consists of a nondisposable syringe with a prefilled, disposable cartridge. This system (Figure 5.60) is becoming increasingly popular because of its ease of operation and speed. The cartridges are packaged in a plastic case, referred to as the Tamp-R-Tel® system (Figure 5.61), that aids in keeping track of controlled medications. Use of the Tubex system follows.

Swing the handle of the syringe downward (Figure 5.62).

Insert a prefilled cartridge (Figure 5.63).

Thread the cartridge into the holder (Figure 5.64).

Thread the plunger onto the cartridge (Figure 5.65).

Expel the air (Figure 5.66).

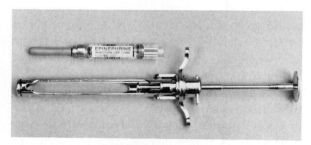

Figure 5.60. The Tubex system.

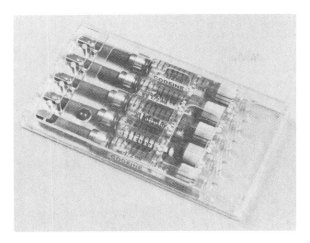

Figure 5.61. The Tamp-R-Tel systems.

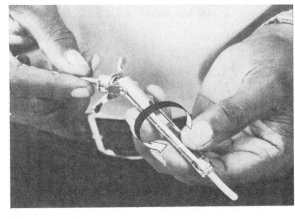

Figure 5.64.

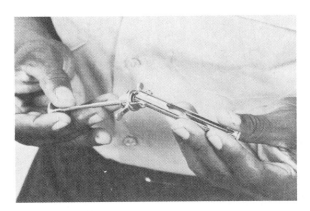

Figure 5.62.

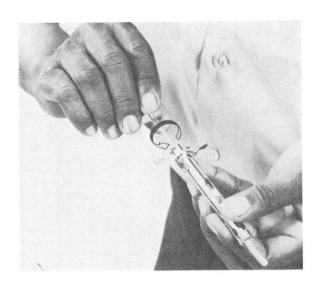

Figure 5.65.

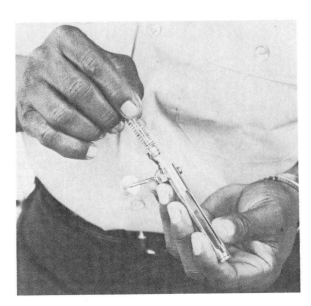

Figure 5.63.

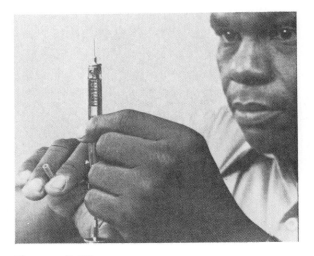

Figure 5.66.

Other Medication Packaging

Many medications used in prehospital care are packaged in the ampules previously described. However, there are other types of medication packaging which may be encountered. The most common of these are the multidose vial and the mix-o-vial system. The technique of preparing an injection from these systems must be slightly modified from that described previously.

MULTIDOSE VIALS

Multidose vials usually contain anywhere from 5 to 30 mL of medication. The required amount is drawn up, and the vial is replaced in stock. The method for withdrawing medication from a vial follows.

Select the appropriate vial (Figure 5.67).

Attach a large-gauge needle (18 gauge) to the syringe (Figure 5.68).

Determine the amount of medication to be administered and withdraw the plunger on the syringe to that amount (Figure 5.69).

Wipe the diaphragm of the vial thoroughly with an alcohol prep (Figure 5.70).

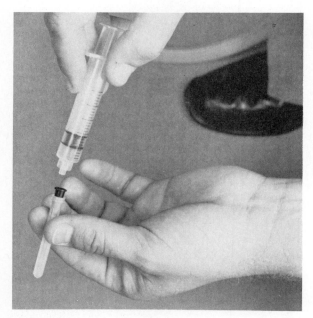

Figure 5.68.

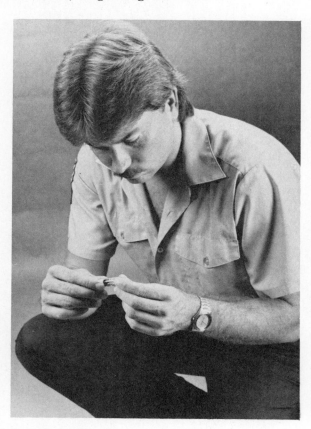

Figure 5.67.

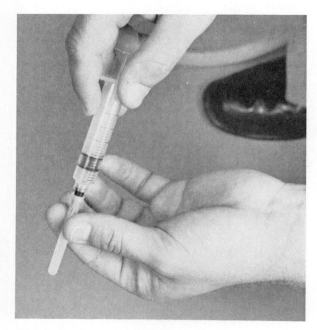

Figure 5.69.

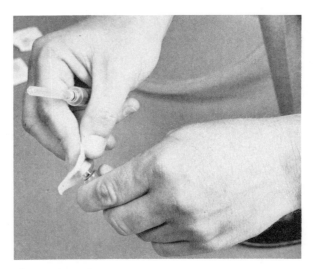

Figure 5.70.

Insert the needle through the diaphragm and depress the plunger forcing the air in the syringe into the vial
(Figure 5.71).

Withdraw the appropriate quantity of
medication (Figure 5.72).

Remove the syringe and recap the
needle (Figure 5.73).

Replace the needle with a smaller needle that will be used for the injection
(Figure 5.74).

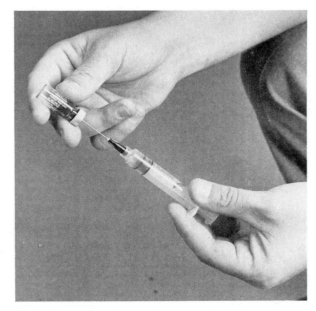

Figure 5.72.

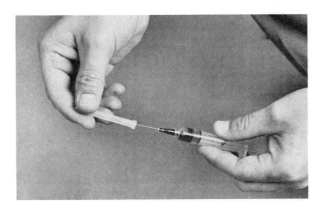

Figure 5.73.

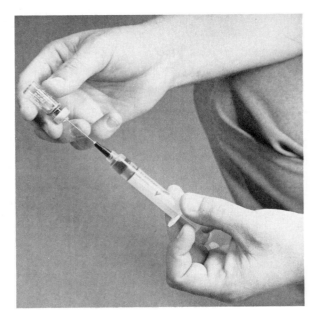

Figure 5.71.

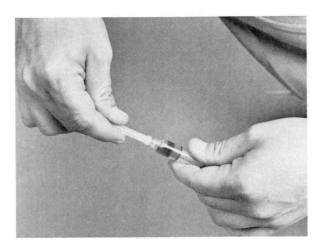

Figure 5.74.

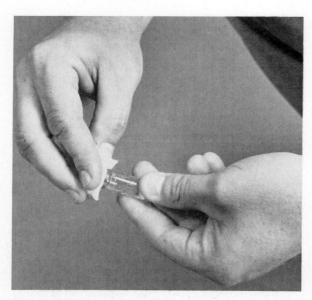

Figure 5.75.

Again, wipe the diaphragm of the vial with an alcohol prep and replace the vial in the drug box (Figure 5.75).

MIX-O-VIAL SYSTEM

The Mix-O-Vial system is used frequently for the packaging of steroid solutions such as methylprednisolone or hydrocortisone.

Prepare a syringe and needle of the appropriate size (Figure 5.76).

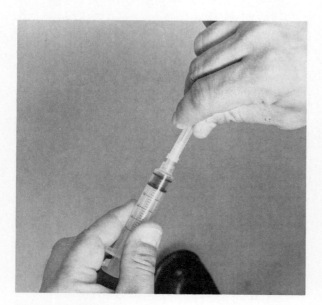

Figure 5.76.

Remove the protective cap from the top of the Mix-O-Vial (Figure 5.77).

Give the plunger–stopper a quarter of a turn and press to force the diluent into lower compartment (Figure 5.78).

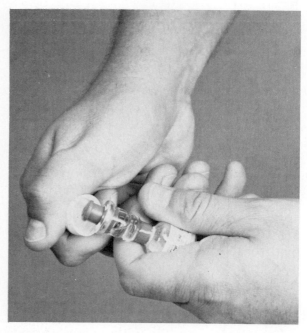

Figure 5.77.

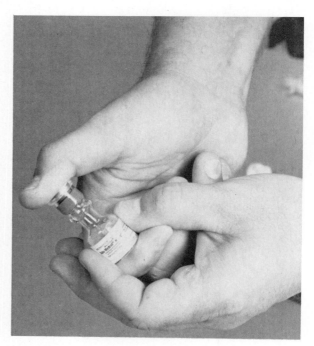

Figure 5.78.

Gently agitate the solution to effect adequate mixing (Figure 5.79).

Insert the needle squarely through the center of the plunger–stopper until the tip is just visible (Figure 5.80). Invert the vial and withdraw the appropriate dose.

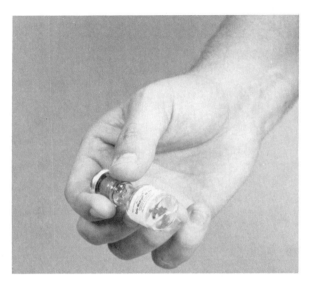

Figure 5.79.

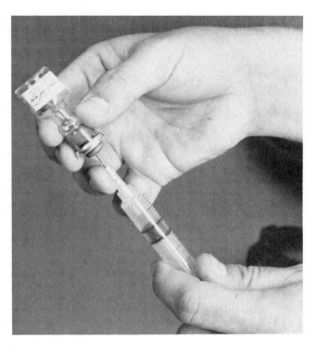

Figure 5.80.

STUDENT NAME _____ **DATE** _____

DIRECTIONS

Evaluate the student by using the criteria presented on this form. Mark PASS for an appropriate action. Mark FAIL for an inappropriate action or missed step. An asterisk (*) indicates an absolute step. Omission of this step indicates automatic failure.

STEP		PASS	FAIL
1.	Prepares the necessary equipment	[ ]	[ ]
2.	Explains procedure to the patient	[ ]	[ ]
3.	Reconfirms patient is not allergic to the medication*	[ ]	[ ]
4.	Selects the correct medication*	[ ]	[ ]
5.	Inspects the medication for discoloration, particles, and checks expiration date	[ ]	[ ]
6.	"Shakes down" the ampule	[ ]	[ ]
7.	Properly breaks the ampule	[ ]	[ ]
8.	Withdraws medication properly	[ ]	[ ]
9.	Chooses appropriate site*	[ ]	[ ]
10.	Preps site with alcohol prep*	[ ]	[ ]
11.	Inserts needle at 90° angle*	[ ]	[ ]
12.	Aspirates for blood*	[ ]	[ ]
13.	Injects medication*	[ ]	[ ]
14.	Applies pressure to site	[ ]	[ ]
15.	Monitors patient and records administration on chart	[ ]	[ ]

TOTAL SCORE (2 points for each PASS)   _____
(20 required for PASS)
NO ABSOLUTES MAY BE FAILED

_____   _____
            Evaluator   Date

Intravenous Drug Administration

Overview

Most medications used in emergency medicine are designed to be administered intravenously. These administrations can be in the form of an IV bolus or as a slow intravenous infusion, sometimes referred to as a piggyback infusion. The rate of absorption is rapid and predictable. However, of all the routes frequently employed in prehospital care, the intravenous administration of drugs has the most potential for causing adverse reactions.

Indications

Intravenous administration is indicated when a fast rate of medication absorption is desired.

Contraindications

Only medications designed for intravenous administration should be administered by this route. You must assure that the dilution and dosage being administered are appropriate for the intravenous route.

Precautions

Assure that the patient is not allergic to the medication you are going to administer. This holds especially true for IV medications because they are introduced directly into the bloodstream and can result in an almost immediate anaphylactic reaction.

IV medications should only be administered through patent, noninfiltrated IVs. Many medications can cause serious tissue damage if extravasated. This statement holds especially true for drugs such as norepinephrine and 50% dextrose in water.

Many medications administered by the intravenous route may interact with other medications being administered at the same time. For example, most of the catecholamines (for example, epinephrine, dopamine, and norepinephrine) are deactivated when mixed with an alkaline solution such as sodium bicarbonate. Calcium chloride and sodium bicarbonate can react together to form a precipitate. This is just a partial list of drug interactions. Because of the possibility of drug interactions, the IV line should always be flushed following the administration of any IV medication to completely eliminate the drug from the tubing.

Complications

Complications from the intravenous administration of medications can occur rapidly and may often be life threatening. The vital signs should be monitored constantly both during and after IV medication administration.

Local complications can also occur. As mentioned previously, extravasation of medications, especially vasoconstrictors and hypertonic solutions, can cause severe tissue necrosis. In addition, pain around the injection site, burning, and edema may sometimes occur.

Intravenous Bolus Administration

Most emergency medications are administered by intravenous bolus. A bolus is a single, oftentimes large, dose of medication given all at once.

Required Equipment

- Medication
- Syringe of adequate size
- Alcohol prep
- 18-gauge Needle

(Many medications used in prehospital care are supplied in a prefilled syringe thus eliminating the need for a separate syringe and needle.)

Procedure

Preload medications for IV administration (Figure 5.81).

Select the appropriate medication (Figure 5.82).

Open the package and remove the contents (Figure 5.83).

Recheck the label on the cartridge and inspect for discoloration or the presence of particles (Figure 5.84).

Remove the caps from medication cartridge and barrel (Figure 5.85).

Engage the syringe (Figure 5.86).

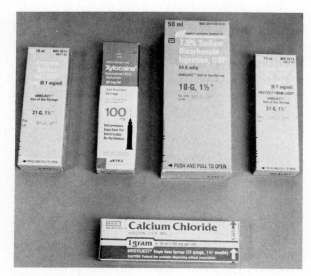

Figure 5.81.

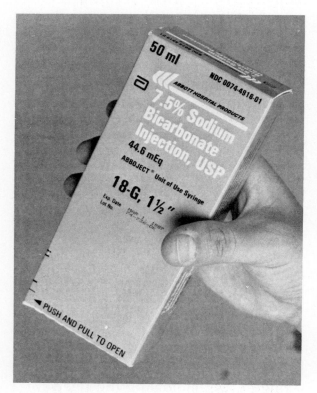

Figure 5.82.

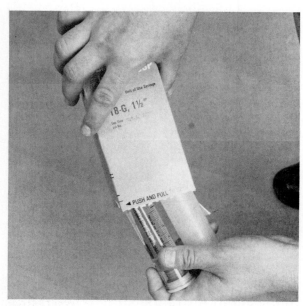

Figure 5.83.

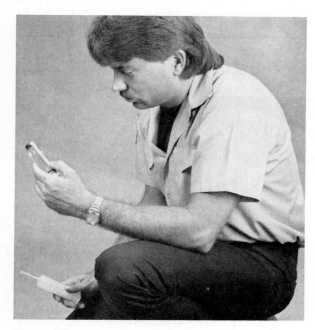

Figure 5.84.

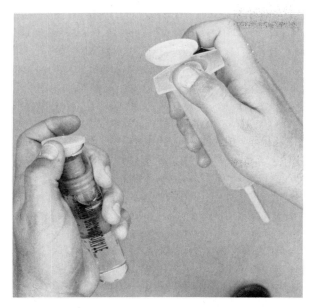

Figure 5.85.

Twist cartridge into the barrel; 3 full turns are usually required (Figure 5.87). Tap the cartridge so as to force the air to the top of the syringe (Figure 5.88). Expel the air (Figure 5.89).

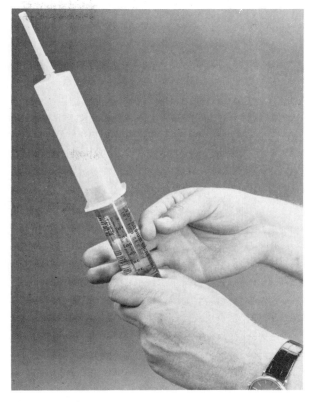

Figure 5.88.

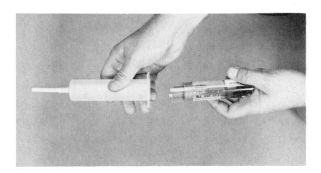

Figure 5.86.

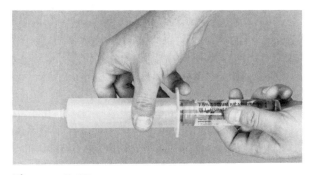

Figure 5.87.

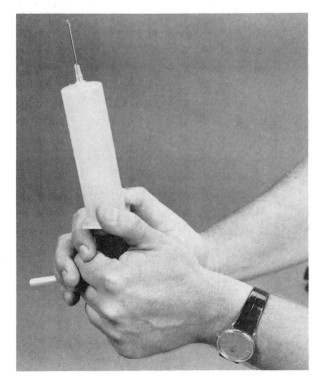

Figure 5.89.

Recap the needle (Figure 5.90).

Prep the medication administration port on the IV tubing with an alcohol prep or another antibacterial solution (Figure 5.91).

Uncap the needle (Figure 5.92).

Insert the needle into the medication administration port (Figure 5.93). Be careful not to push the needle through the other side of the port.

Pinch the tubing above the medication port to prevent the drug from flowing back into the IV bag (Figure 5.94).

Inject the medication in a deliberate fashion (Figure 5.95). Some medications, such as 50% dextrose in water, take considerably longer to inject than others.

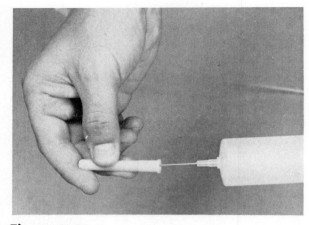

Figure 5.92.

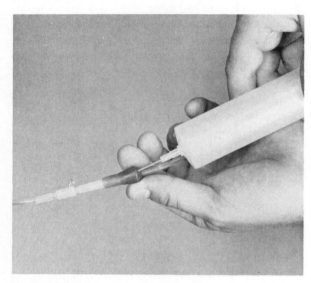

Figure 5.93.

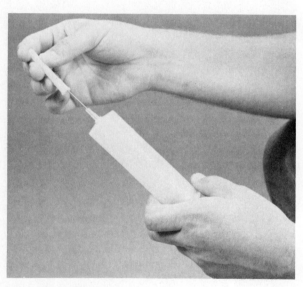

Figure 5.90.

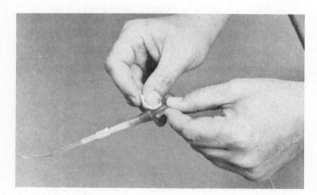

Figure 5.91.

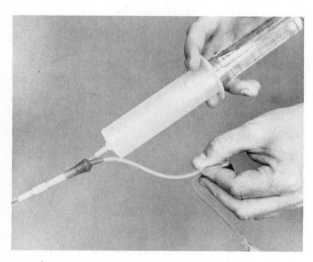

Figure 5.94.

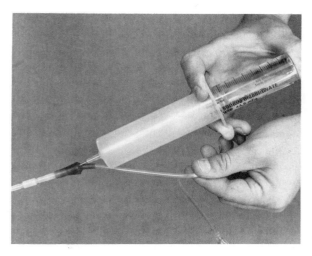

Figure 5.95.

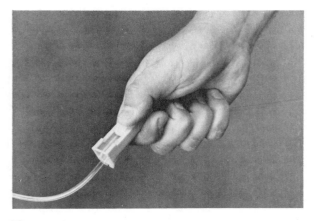

Figure 5.97.

Remove the needle, recap, and place in a safe place (Figure 5.96).

Open the IV control valve to flush the line to completely eliminate the medication from the tubing (Figure 5.97).

Record the time and dosage administered on the patient report (Figure 5.98).

Monitor the patient for the desired effects as well as for any adverse reactions (Figure 5.99).

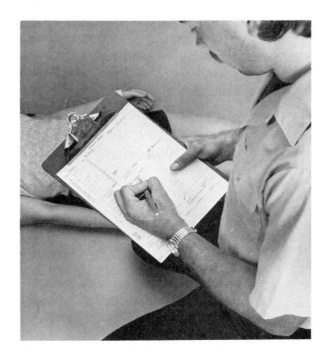

Figure 5.98.

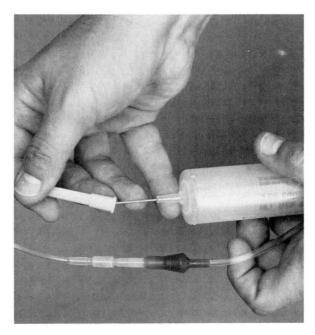

Figure 5.96.

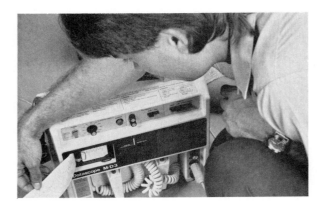

Figure 5.99.

STUDENT NAME _____ **DATE** _____

DIRECTIONS

Evaluate the student by using the criteria presented on this form. Mark PASS for an appropriate action. Mark FAIL for an inappropriate action or missed step. An asterisk (*) indicates an absolute step. Omission of this step indicates automatic failure.

	STEP	PASS	FAIL
1.	Prepares the necessary equipment	[ ]	[ ]
2.	Reconfirms that the patient is not allergic to the medication*	[ ]	[ ]
3.	Selects the correct medication*	[ ]	[ ]
4.	Inspects medication for discoloration, particles, and checks expiration date	[ ]	[ ]
5.	Assembles the prefilled syringe	[ ]	[ ]
6.	Expels air from the syringe*	[ ]	[ ]
7.	Cleanses medication administration port with alcohol prep*	[ ]	[ ]
8.	Inserts needle into port*	[ ]	[ ]
9.	Pinches tubing above the port*	[ ]	[ ]
10.	Injects the correct amount of medication*	[ ]	[ ]
11.	Removes needle and recaps syringe	[ ]	[ ]
12.	Opens IV control valve to flush the line	[ ]	[ ]
13.	Records the administration	[ ]	[ ]
14.	Monitors the patient for desired effects*	[ ]	[ ]

TOTAL SCORE (2 points for each PASS)   _____
(20 required for PASS)
NO ABSOLUTES MAY BE FAILED

Evaluator _____   Date _____

Intravenous Infusion (Piggyback Infusion)

Several IV medications are designed to be administered by a slow intravenous infusion. Common medications used in the prehospital setting administered in this fashion include lidocaine, procainamide, dopamine, isoproterenol, and norepinephrine. Most of these medications are used for long-term support of heart rate, blood pressure, or for the suppression of arrhythmias.

Medications administered by the piggyback route often must be diluted before they can be administered. The dilution used for the medications just listed varies from region to region.

Medications should not be added to the original IV infusion. Many medica-

tions used for IV infusions are supplied in prefilled syringes designed for easy addition to the IV bag or bottle.

Required Equipment

- Medication
- Syringe
- 18-gauge Needles (2)
- Alcohol prep
- Label
- 5% Dextrose in water (D5W) (for dilution)
- 1-inch Tape
- Minidrip administration set

Procedure

Required equipment (Figure 5.100).
Prefilled medication for dilution (Figure 5.101).
Select the medication (Figure 5.102).

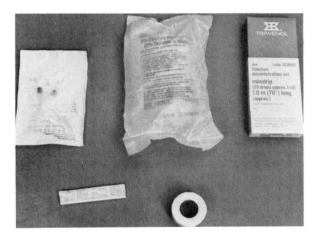

Figure 5.100.

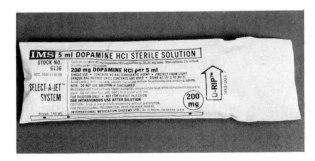

Figure 5.101.

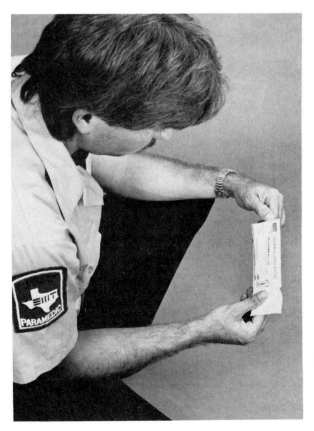

Figure 5.102.

Select a bag of 5% dextrose in water of appropriate quantity for dilution (Figure 5.103).

Inspect the medication for discoloration or for the presence of particles (Figure 5.104).

Assemble the syringe (Figure 5.105).

Inject medication into the bag (Figure 5.106).

Invert the bag several times to mix the medication (Figure 5.107).

Insert minidrip administration set (Figure 5.108).

Connect the needle to the administration set (Figure 5.109).

Squeeze the drip chamber (Figure 5.110).

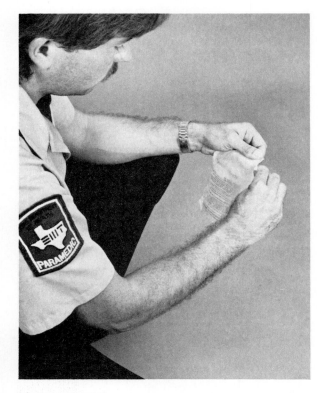

Figure 5.104.

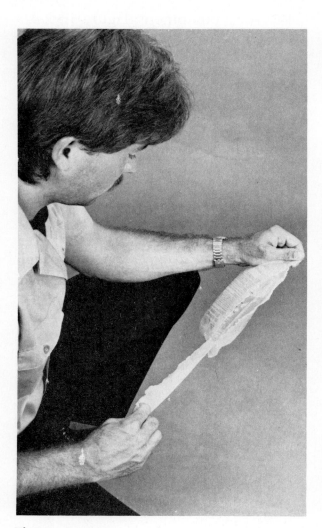

Figure 5.103.

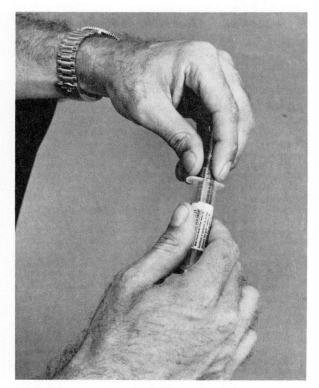

Figure 5.105.

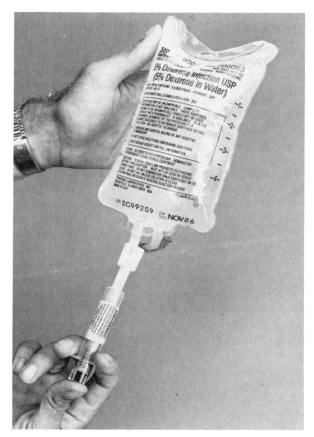

Figure 5.106.

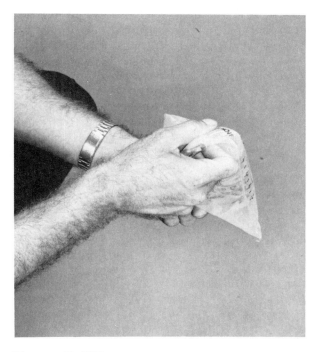

Figure 5.107.

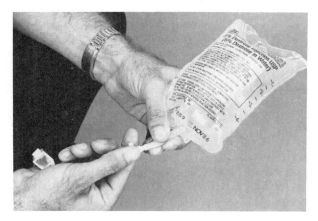

Figure 5.108.

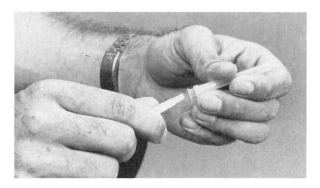

Figure 5.109.

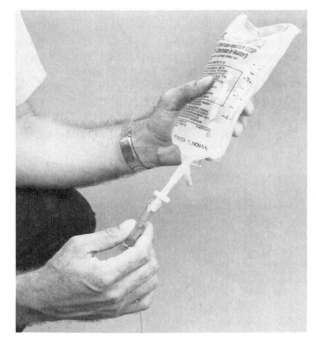

Figure 5.110.

Flush the IV line (Figure 5.111).

Prep the IV medication port on the first IV administration set (Figure 5.112)

Insert the piggyback needle into the medication port (Figure 5.113).

Securely tape the needle in place (Figure 5.114).

Set infusion at the desired rate (Figure 5.115).

Label the bag with the name of the drug, the dilution, the time administration was started, and your initials (Figure 5.116).

Note administration of the drug on the patient report (Figure 5.117).

Monitor patient for the desired effects and any possible adverse reactions (Figure 5.118).

When more than one piggyback infusion is in place each IV tube should be labeled (Figure 5.119).

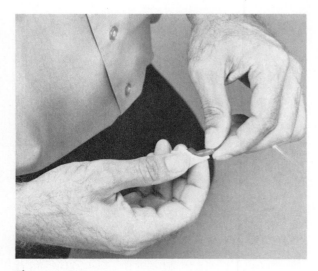

Figure 5.112.

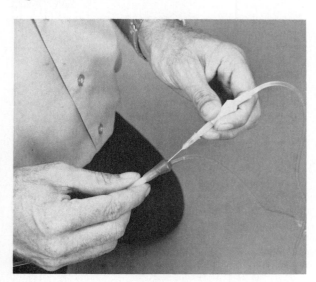

Figure 5.113.

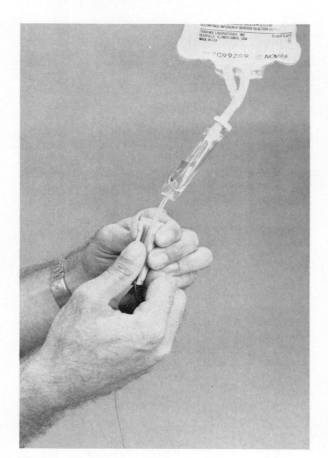

Figure 5.111.

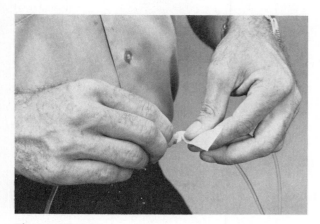

Figure 5.114.

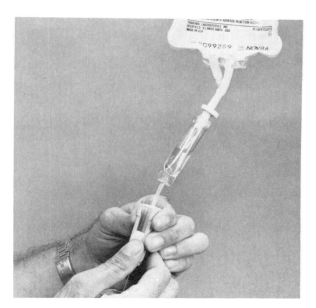

Figure 5.115.

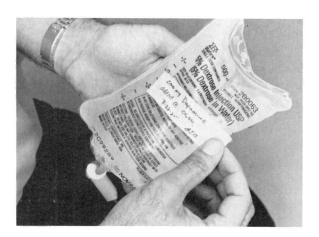

Figure 5.116.

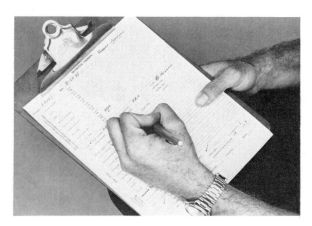

Figure 5.117.

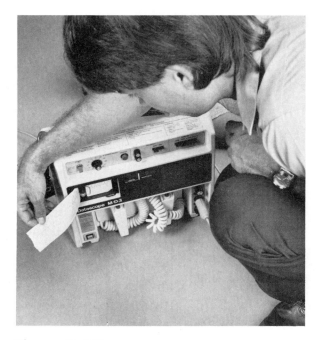

Figure 5.118.

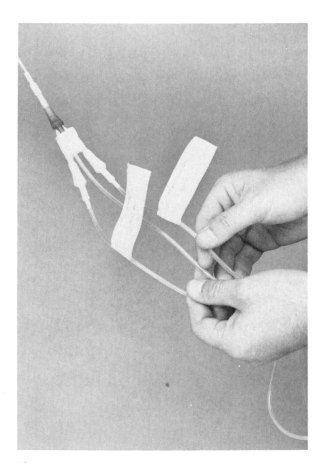

Figure 5.119.

STUDENT NAME ———————————————————————— **DATE** ——————————

DIRECTIONS

Evaluate the student by using the criteria presented on this form. Mark PASS for an appropriate action. Mark FAIL for an inappropriate action or missed step. An asterisk (*) indicates an absolute step. Omission of this step indicates automatic failure.

STEP	PASS	FAIL

IV PIGGYBACK ADMINISTRATION

	STEP	PASS	FAIL
1.	Prepare the necessary equipment	[ ]	[ ]
2.	Reconfirms that the patient is not allergic to the medication*	[ ]	[ ]
3.	Selects the correct medication*	[ ]	[ ]
4.	Inspects the medication for discoloration, particles, and checks expiration date	[ ]	[ ]
5.	Cleanses medication addition port*	[ ]	[ ]
6.	Properly adds the medication to the proper IV fluid (D5W)	[ ]	[ ]
7.	Mixes the solution by inverting the bag several times	[ ]	[ ]
8.	Connects the administration set by using aseptic technique	[ ]	[ ]
9.	Flushes IV line and expels any air present	[ ]	[ ]
10.	Attaches needle to piggyback line	[ ]	[ ]
11.	Cleanses medication administration port and inserts needle*	[ ]	[ ]
12.	Secures needle	[ ]	[ ]
13.	Sets infusion at desired rate*	[ ]	[ ]
14.	Labels the bag appropriately	[ ]	[ ]
15.	Monitors the patient for desired effects	[ ]	[ ]

TOTAL SCORE (2 points for each PASS) ————————
(21 required for PASS)
NO ABSOLUTES MAY BE FAILED

————————————————————————————— —————————————————
Evaluator   Date

Blood Glucose Analysis Using Dextrostix® Reagent Strips

Overview

Approximate blood glucose levels can be determined rapidly by using Dextrostix reagent strips. This simple test is extremely useful when treating suspected diabetics or patients with a coma of unknown origin. The test takes only one minute to complete and requires as little as 1 mL of blood.

Indications

1. Diabetic emergencies
2. Coma of unknown origin

Contraindications

None when used in the situations just described.

Precautions

Remember that Dextrostix only approximates the blood glucose level. Significant variations in the reading may result from out of date reagent strips, overdeveloping or underdeveloping of the test, or from using a contaminated wash solution. Dextrostix should NEVER be washed with a dextrose solution such as 5% dextrose in water.

Complications

An inaccurate test may result in improper or delayed treatment. Follow the directions specifically and adhere to the recommended exposure times.

Required Equipment

- Dextrostix reagent strips
- Vacutainer barrel
- Red top vacutainer tube
- Watch

- Band-Aid
- Vacutainer needles
- Antiseptic solution
- Water in wash bottle
- 2×2 Gauze pad

Procedure

Check the expiration date on the Dextrostix reagent strip package (Figure 5.120).

Prepare the equipment (Figure 5.121).

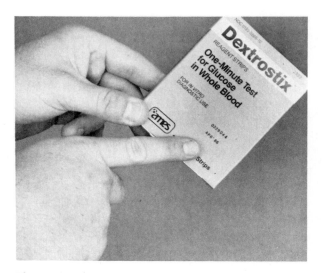

Figure 5.120.

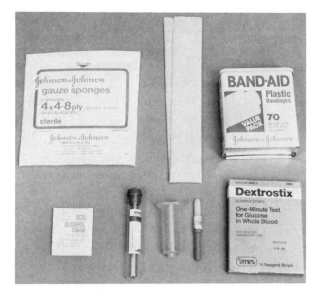

Figure 5.121.

Insert the needle onto the Vacutainer barrel and loosely insert the Vacutainer tube (Figure 5.122).

Apply the venous constricting band, select a suitable vein, and apply antiseptic solution (Figure 5.123).

Enter the vein and fill the Vacutainer tube with blood (Figure 5.124).

Remove the needle from the vein and cover the puncture site with a gauze pad (Figure 5.125).

Allow a drop or two of blood to drip onto reagent portion of Dextrostix reagent strip (Figure 5.126). NOTE THE TIME.

Wait exactly 60 seconds before washing the reagent strip (Figure 5.127).

After 60 seconds has passed, thoroughly wash the reagent portion of the Dextrostix with water (Figure 5.128).

Immediately compare the color of the reagent strip to the color chart on the Dextrostix packaging material (Figure 5.129).

Note the approximate blood glucose reading on the patient report form (Figure 5.130).

Label the Vacutainer tube with the patient's name, time, date, and your initials (Figure 5.131).

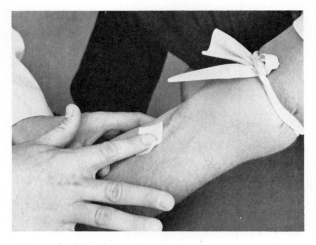

Figure 5.123.

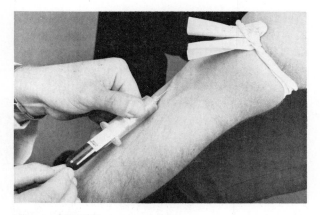

Figure 5.124.

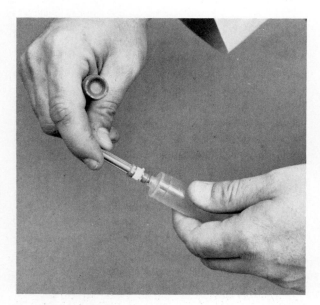

Figure 5.122.

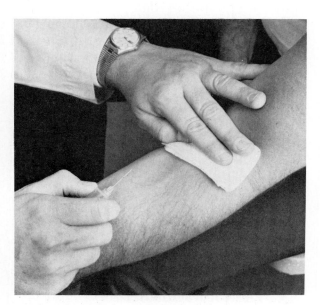

Figure 5.125.

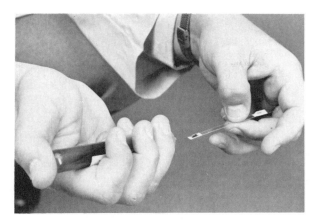

Figure 5.126.

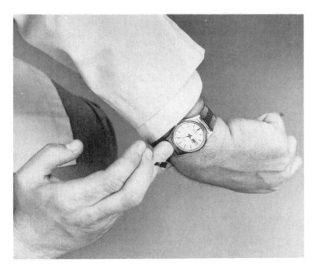

Figure 5.127.

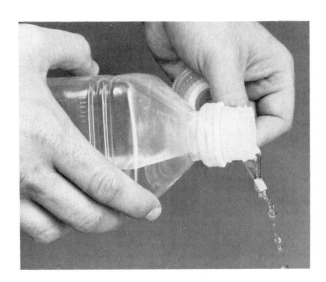

Figure 5.128.

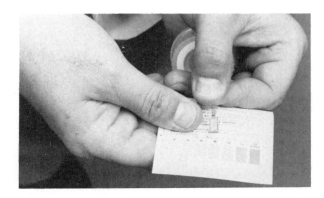

Figure 5.129.

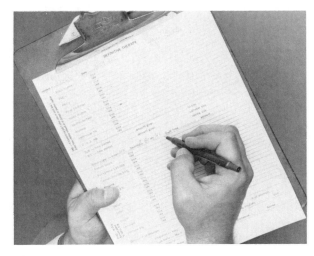

Figure 5.130.

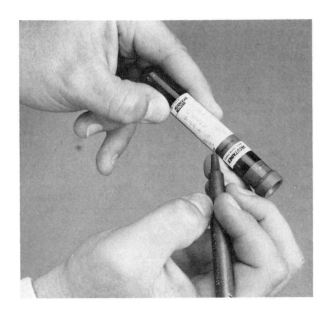

Figure 5.131.

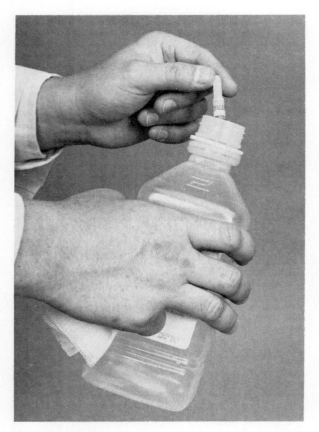

Figure 5.132.

Properly dispose of all expended materials (Figure 5.132).

Alternate Technique

Instead of using the vacutainer barrel system, the blood sample may be taken while inserting an indwelling cannula. This is done by attaching a 5 mL syringe to the indwelling cannula after the vein has been entered and withdrawing approximately 5 mL of blood.

Make the puncture with an indwelling cannula and withdraw approximately 5 mL of blood. (Figure 5.133).

Attach the IV line and begin infusion (Figure 5.134).

Place an 18-gauge needle on the syringe and insert it into the red top tube (Figure 5.135).

Allow the blood to enter the tube (Figure 5.136). Do not try and force the blood into the tube. The vacuum pre-

sent in the tube will allow only a set quantity of blood to enter the tube.

With the blood remaining in the syringe perform a blood glucose analysis as just described (Figure 5.137).

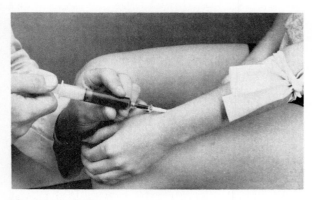

Figure 5.133.

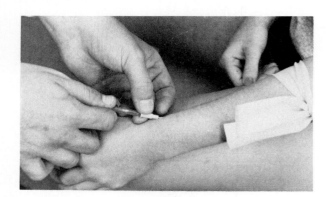

Figure 5.134.

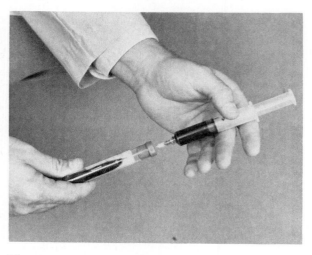

Figure 5.135.

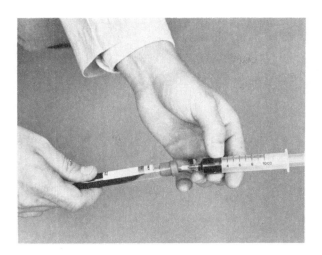

Figure 5.136.

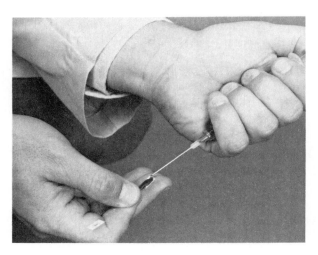

Figure 5.137.

STUDENT NAME ———————————————————————— **DATE** ——————————

DIRECTIONS

Evaluate the student by using the criteria presented on this form. Mark PASS for an appropriate action. Mark FAIL for an inappropriate action or missed step. An asterisk (*) indicates an absolute step. Omission of this step indicates automatic failure.

STEP	PASS	FAIL

BLOOD GLUCOSE ANALYSIS USING DEXTROSTIX REAGENT STRIPS

	STEP	PASS	FAIL
1.	Prepares the necessary equipment	[ ]	[ ]
2.	Checks expiration date*	[ ]	[ ]
3.	Assembles vacutainer syringe	[ ]	[ ]
4.	Applies tourniquet and chooses a suitable vein	[ ]	[ ]
5.	Cleanses puncture site with antibacterial solution*	[ ]	[ ]
6.	Enters the vein and withdraws a tube of blood	[ ]	[ ]
7.	Places a drop of blood on Dextrostix reagent strip and notes time*	[ ]	[ ]
8.	Waits 60 seconds*	[ ]	[ ]
9.	Washes Dextrostix with water	[ ]	[ ]
10.	Immediately reads results	[ ]	[ ]
11.	Notes results on patient report form	[ ]	[ ]
12.	Labels tube with blood	[ ]	[ ]
13.	Properly disposes of expended materials	[ ]	[ ]

TOTAL SCORE (2 points for each PASS) ————————
(18 required for PASS)
NO ABSOLUTES MAY BE FAILED

——————————————————————————— ————————————————————
Evaluator   Date

Transtracheal Medication Instillation

Overview

The transtracheal route of drug administration is very effective and is often forgotten in the emergency setting. When an IV cannot be established, and the patient is in dire need of lidocaine, atropine, or epinephrine, which may be the case in cardiac arrest, these drugs may be instilled via a properly placed endotracheal tube. These drugs are absorbed by the pulmonary capillaries and quickly reach the target organ. The rate of absorption of drugs administered transtracheally is as fast as IV administration. Transtracheal administration is preferred over the intracardiac route.

Indications

Transtracheal administration is indicated in patients in whom an IV line cannot be initiated and who require either lidocaine, epinephrine, or atropine.

Contraindications

Transtracheal administration should only be used for the three drugs just listed unless otherwise directed by your medical director.

Precautions

To prevent hypoxia, the patient must be hyperventilated before removing the bag–valve–mask unit and injecting the medication.

No more than 10 mL of a drug should be administered transtracheally.

Complications

Drugs administered by the transtracheal route may be ineffective if the patient has aspirated large amounts of material or is experiencing severe pulmonary edema.

Required Equipment

- Medication
- Needle
- Syringe

Procedure

Select the appropriate medication (Figure 5.138).

Open the package and examine the drug for discoloration or the presence of particles (Figure 5.139).

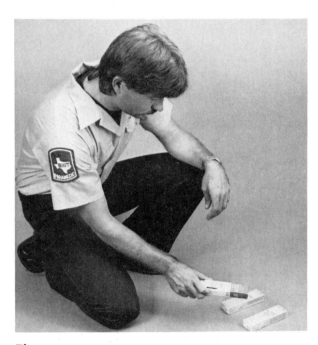

Figure 5.138.

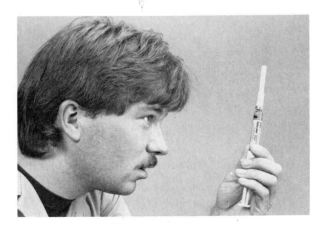

Figure 5.139.

Hyperventilate the patient in anticipation of drug administration (Figure 5.140).

Remove the bag–valve–mask unit and inject the medication down the tube (Figure 5.141).

Replace the bag–valve–mask (BVM) unit and resume ventilations (Figure 5.142).

Monitor the patient for the desired therapeutic effects as well as for any possible undesired side effects (Figure 5.143).

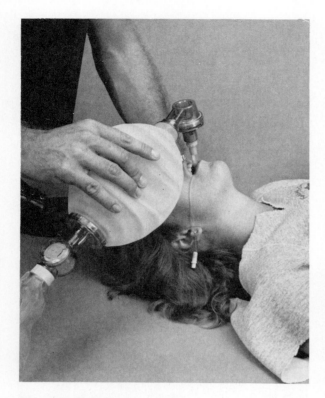

Figure 5.140.

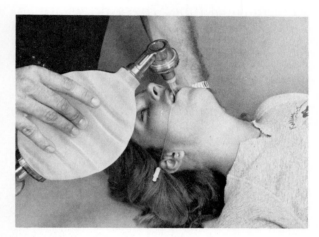

Figure 5.142.

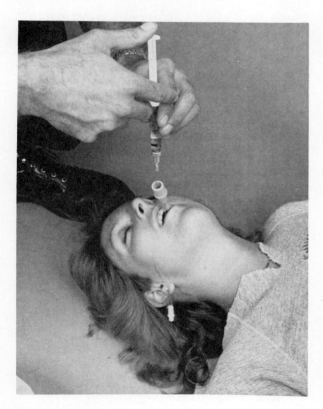

Figure 5.141.

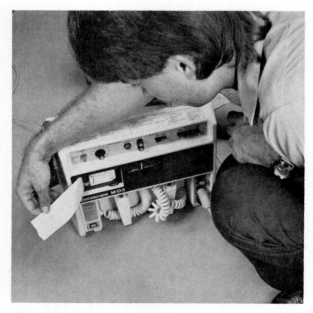

Figure 5.143.

STUDENT NAME _____ **DATE** _____

DIRECTIONS

Evaluate the student by using the criteria presented on this form. Mark PASS for an appropriate action. Mark FAIL for an inappropriate action or missed step. An asterisk (*) indicates an absolute step. Omission of this step indicates automatic failure.

STEP	PASS	FAIL
TRANSTRACHEAL MEDICATION ADMINISTRATION		
1. Receives the order	[ ]	[ ]
2. Prepares the necessary equipment	[ ]	[ ]
3. Examines the medication for discoloration or the presence of particles*	[ ]	[ ]
4. Assembles the syringe	[ ]	[ ]
5. Hyperventilates the patient in anticipation of administration*	[ ]	[ ]
6. Removes the BVM and administers the medication	[ ]	[ ]
7. Replaces the BVM and resumes ventilation	[ ]	[ ]
8. Monitors the patient for the desired effects*	[ ]	[ ]

TOTAL SCORE (2 points for each PASS)   _____
(11 required for PASS)
NO ABSOLUTES MAY BE FAILED

_____ _____
Evaluator　　　　　　　　　　Date

Intracardiac Medication Administration

Overview

Injection of medication directly into the ventricle of the heart is referred to as intracardiac administration. Intracardiac injection was employed for many years as a primary route of medication administration in treating cardiac arrest. In recent years, however, transtracheal and intravenous administration of emergency medications have been found to be just as effective and much less dangerous than the intracardiac route. Because of the possible complications inherent in this procedure, it is reserved for use only in those cases where an IV cannot be established or an endotracheal tube cannot be placed.

There are two accepted approaches to intracardiac medication injection. One method, the subxiphoid approach (Figure 5.144), involves inserting the needle into the chest at the left inferior costal border and advancing the needle toward the left shoulder and into the ventricle.

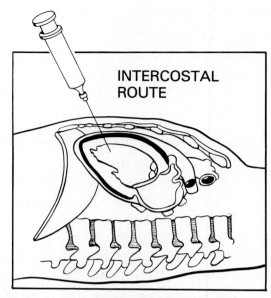

Figure 5.145. Intercostal approach to intracardiac medication administration.

The other method, the intercostal approach (Figure 5.145), involves inserting the needle through the fourth intercostal space and into the ventricle. Generally, the subxiphoid approach is preferred as the likelihood of injuring the coronary arteries is minimal.

Indications

Cardiac arrest where an IV cannot be established or an endotracheal tube cannot be placed.

Contraindications

No relevant contraindications exist when used in the situation just described.

Precautions

It is important to determine that the ventricle has been entered as evidenced by signficant blood return before injecting the medication. Injection of medications into the myocardium can result in considerable muscle damage.

Most medications used for intracardiac injection (epinephrine and calcium chloride) come with an intracardiac nee-

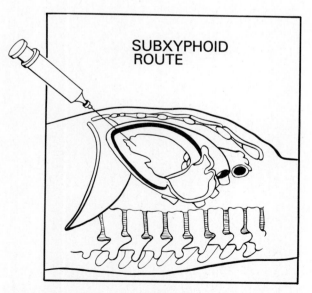

Figure 5.144. Subxiphoid approach to intracardiac medication administration.

dle already attached to the prefilled syringe. Usually these needles are for adult intracardiac administration and should not be used for pediatric cases.

Complications

Possible complications include accidental laceration of the coronary arteries, intramyocardial injection, intraseptal injection, pericardial tamponade, and pneumothorax.

Required Equipment

- Medication (epinephrine or calcium chloride)
- Syringe (usually prefilled)
- 3-inch needle (spinal needle)
- Antibacterial prep

Procedure

Uncap the syringe (Figure 5.146).
Expel any air present (Figure 5.147).
Palpate the left subcostal border (Figure 5.148).
Prep the area with an antibacterial solution (Figure 5.149).

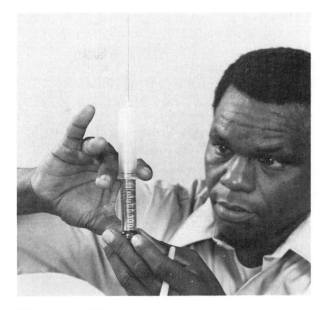

Figure 5.147.

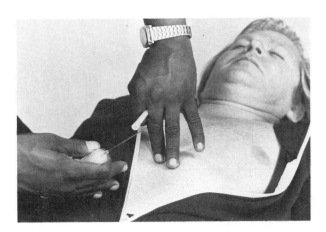

Figure 5.148.

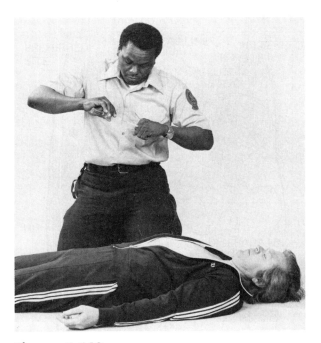

Figure 5.146.

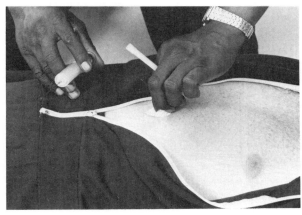

Figure 5.149.

Insert the needle and advance toward the left shoulder (Figure 5.150). Use caution not to touch the needle with an ungloved hand.

Aspirate for free blood (Figure 5.151). The presence of free blood indicates entry into the ventricle.

Inject the medication (Figure 5.152).

Remove the needle and massage the injection site with firm pressure (Figure 5.153).

Resume CPR and monitor for the effects of the medication (Figure 5.154).

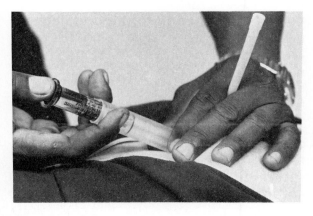

Figure 5.152.

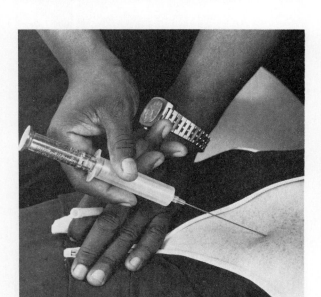

Figure 5.150.

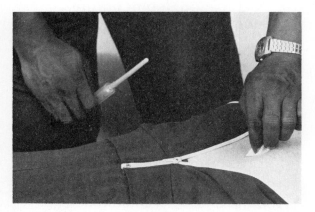

Figure 5.153.

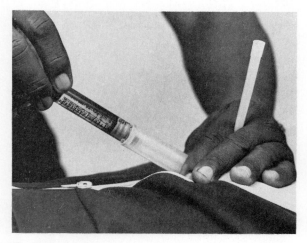

Figure 5.151.

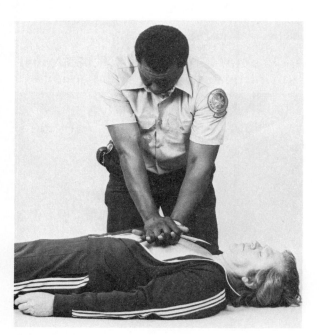

Figure 5.154.

STUDENT NAME _____ **DATE** _____

DIRECTIONS

Evaluate the student by using the criteria presented on this form. Mark PASS for an appropriate action. Mark FAIL for an inappropriate action or missed step. An asterisk (*) indicates an absolute step. Omission of this step indicates automatic failure.

STEP	PASS	FAIL

INTRACARDIAC MEDICATION ADMINISTRATION

	STEP	PASS	FAIL
1.	Receives the order	[ ]	[ ]
2.	Prepares the necessary equipment	[ ]	[ ]
3.	Examines the medication for discoloration or the presence of particles*	[ ]	[ ]
4.	Assembles the syringe	[ ]	[ ]
5.	Palpates the left subcostal border*	[ ]	[ ]
6.	Preps the area with an antibacterial solution	[ ]	[ ]
7.	Stops CPR	[ ]	[ ]
8.	Inserts the needle and advances toward the left shoulder	[ ]	[ ]
9.	Aspirates for blood*	[ ]	[ ]
10.	Injects the medication	[ ]	[ ]
11.	Removes needle and massages the injection site*	[ ]	[ ]
12.	Resumes CPR*	[ ]	[ ]
13.	Monitors for the effects of the medication*	[ ]	[ ]

TOTAL SCORE (2 points for each PASS) _____
(18 required for PASS)
NO ABSOLUTES MAY BE FAILED

_____   _____
            Evaluator   Date

Nitronox Administration

Overview

Nitronox is a blended mixture of 50% nitrous oxide and 50% oxygen. When inhaled, it has potent analgesic effects. These effects, however, quickly dissipate within 2–5 minutes after cessation of administration. This makes Nitronox an ideal analgesic for use in prehospital care.

The Nitronox unit consists of one oxygen and one nitrous oxide cylinder (Figure 5.155). The gases are fed from these cylinders into a blender which combines them at the appropriate (50%/50%) concentration. The mixed gas is then deliv-

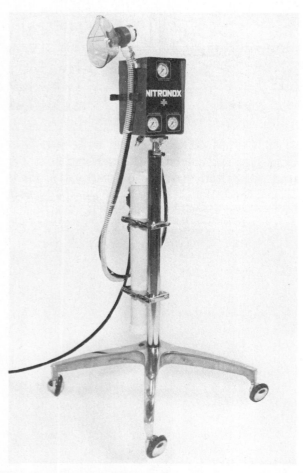

Figure 5.155. Nitronox unit for inhospital use.

ered to a modified demand valve for administration to the patient.

Nitronox should always be self-administered and is effective for treating most varieties of pain encountered in emergency medicine, including the pain accompanying various forms of trauma. The high concentration of oxygen delivered along with the nitrous oxide will aid in increasing oxygen tension in the blood, thus reducing hypoxia.

Indications

Moderate to severe pain.

Contraindications

Nitronox is contraindicated in patients with severe head injury as it can cause an increase in intracranial pressure.

Precautions

It is essential that Nitronox be self-administered if possible. Also, nitrous oxide may cause vomiting in susceptible individuals which should be anticipated.

Prolonged use of the device will sometimes cause icing of the nitrous oxide cylinder head and the associated lines.

Complications

No major complications appear to be associated with the use of Nitronox as long as it is self-administered by the patient. The device is designed to shut down when the oxygen supply is depleted. However, the device will continue to deliver oxygen when the nitrous oxide is depleted.

Some patients may experience hallucinations or bizarre thoughts while under the influence of Nitronox.

Required Equipment

- Nitronox unit
- Nitrous oxide
- Oxygen
- Cylinder wrench

Procedure

Receive the order (Figure 5.156).

Open the case and open both the oxygen and nitrous oxide cylinders (Figure 5.157).

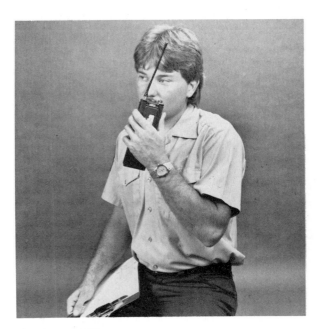

Figure 5.156.

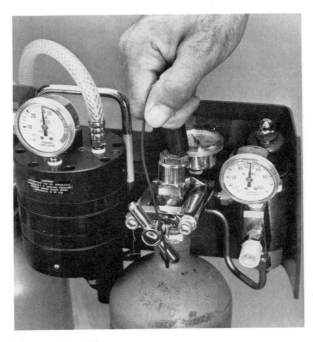

Figure 5.157.

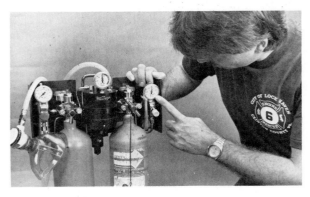

Figure 5.158.

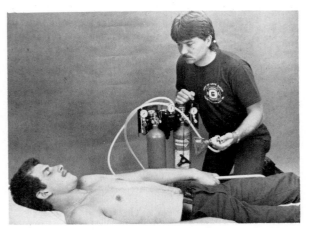

Figure 5.159.

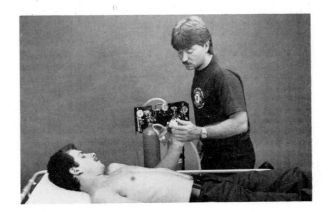

Figure 5.160.

Check cylinder pressures and line pressure (Figure 5.158).

Remove the demand valve from its storage position (Figure 5.159).

Instruct the patient on the use of the device (Figure 5.160).

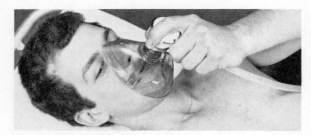

Figure 5.161.

Allow the patient to breathe through the demand valve (Figure 5.161).

Monitor the patient's level of consciousness and degree of analgesia (Figure 5.162).

Be prepared to maintain the patient's airway if the patient drops the mask or becomes unconscious (Figure 5.163).

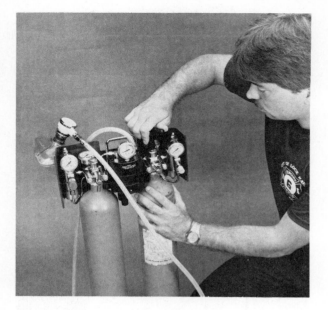

Figure 5.164.

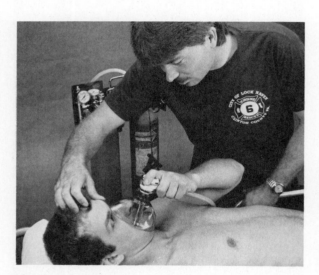

Figure 5.162.

Following Administration

After administration, note the pressure remaining in both cylinders (Figure 5.164). Close both cylinders.

Clean the mask and return it to its storage position (Figure 5.165).

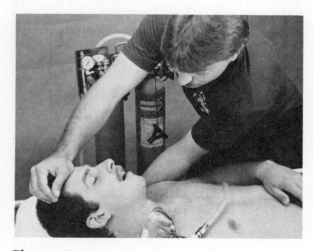

Figure 5.163.

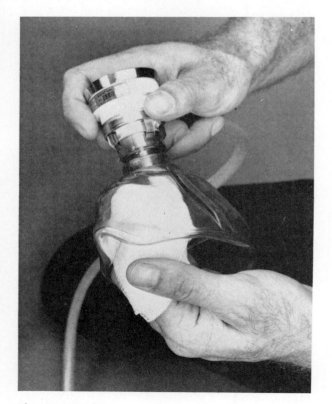

Figure 5.165.

STUDENT NAME _____ **DATE** _____

DIRECTIONS

Evaluate the student by using the criteria presented on this form. Mark PASS for an appropriate action. Mark FAIL for an inappropriate action or missed step. An asterisk (*) indicates an absolute step. Omission of this step indicates automatic failure.

STEP	PASS	FAIL
NITRONOX ADMINISTRATION		
1. Receives the order	[ ]	[ ]
2. Opens the case and turns on both the oxygen and nitrous oxide cylinders	[ ]	[ ]
3. Checks pressure in each cylinder	[ ]	[ ]
4. Checks line pressure	[ ]	[ ]
5. Removes and inspects the mask	[ ]	[ ]
6. Explains to patient how to use the device.*	[ ]	[ ]
7. Allows the patient to breathe through the demand valve	[ ]	[ ]
8. Monitors the patient's level of consciousness*	[ ]	[ ]
9. After administration, notes the remaining pressure	[ ]	[ ]
10. Closes both cylinders and cleans the mask	[ ]	[ ]

TOTAL SCORE (2 points for each PASS) _____
(14 required for PASS)
NO ABSOLUTES MAY BE FAILED

_____ | _____
Evaluator | Date

Nasogastric Tube Insertion

Overview

A nasogastric tube is a tube that is placed through the nose, down the esophagus, and into the stomach. Nasogastric tubes are frequently inserted in the emergency department and are occasionally inserted in the prehospital setting. Nasogastric intubation is performed primarily to: remove stomach contents (air, food, etc.), to dilute or wash out (lavage) ingested poisons, and to remove blood in cases of gastrointestinal (GI) hemorrhage with subsequent washing with iced saline.

Three types of nasogastric tubes are used in emergency medicine, the Ewald, Levin, or Salem Sump. The tubes are supplied in various sizes. Levin and Salem Sump tubes are generally 12-18 French, while the Ewald (red rubber) is used in 32-36 French sizes. The Ewald tube is used for rapid lavage of gastric contents.

Indications

Nasogastric intubation is indicated in cases where evacuation or lavage of the stomach contents is ordered. Gastric lavage is preferably deferred until the patient is in the emergency department. However, it is recognized that there are many EMS systems with extremely long transport times where prehospital gastric lavage may be helpful or even lifesaving.

Contraindications

Patients with severe facial trauma, that especially involves the nasal area, should have nasogastric intubation deferred until they are in the emergency department.

Nasogastric intubation should not be attempted, in the prehospital phase of emergency care, in patients with epiglottitis or croup (laryngotracheobron-

chitis) as the presence of the tube may induce vocal cord spasm.

Precautions

The patient must understand the procedure, if conscious, and be instructed to mouth-breathe and swallow as the tube is passed. It is best to have the patient semi-sitting if his condition permits. Dentures should be removed. The nasal passages should be inspected prior to attempting nasogastric intubation. Patients with a significantly deviated nasal septum or with significant nasal obstructions should have nasogastric intubation deferred until they are in the emergency department.

The nasogastric tube, and sometimes the nostril itself, should be well lubricated with a water-soluble lubricant such as K-Y jelly.

It may be difficult to insert a nasogastric tube in the patient who has an endotracheal tube in place. If the tube will not pass into the stomach because of the inflated endotracheal tube cuff in the trachea, then the cuff can be deflated long enough for passage of the nasogastric tube. Regardless, the airway must be protected, and suction should be readily available.

Attempts to pass a nasogastric tube in conscious patients will almost always result in elicitation of the gag reflex. If the patient starts to gag, stop insertion of the tube and allow the patient to take a few deep breaths before you continue. Sometimes it is necessary to allow the patient to take a few sips of water as the tube is passed from the nasopharynx into the esophagus.

Complications

Epistaxis is a common complication of nasogastric intubation. It frequently occurs when too large a tube is used or if the tube is not adequately lubricated. It is not uncommon for the tube to curl up inside the pharynx as intubation is attempted. If this occurs, the tube should be withdrawn and intubation reattempted.

Insertion of the tube into the trachea is possible. If breath sounds are heard through the tube, or if the patient begins coughing, gasping, or becomes cyanotic, then withdraw the tube and attempt reinsertion. If you are unsure of the placement of the tube you can immerse the end of the tube in a glass of water. If bubbles appear upon expiration the tube is improperly placed in the trachea.

Required Equipment

- Levin or Salem Sump tube (16-18 French for adults)
- 50-mL Syringe with plain tip
- Water-soluble lubricant
- Adhesive tape
- Saline for irrigation
- Drinking water with straw

Procedure

Required equipment (Figure 5.166).

Prepare equipment (Figure 5.167). Be sure to adequately lubricate 6–8 inches of the distal tube.

Mark the distance the tube should be inserted by measuring the distance from the ear lobe to the bridge of the nose and then from the bridge of the nose to below the xiphoid process. Mark the point on the tube (Figure 5.168).

Examine the nose for septal deviation (Figure 5.169).

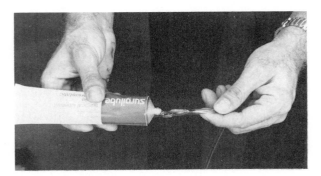

Figure 5.167.

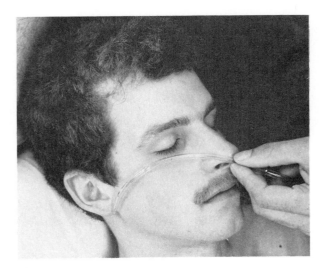

Figure 5.168.

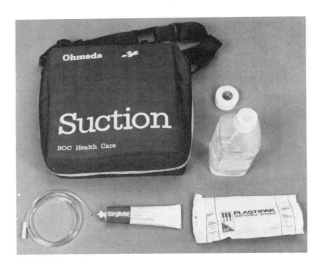

Figure 5.166.

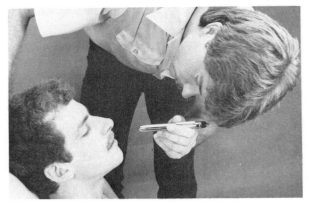

Figure 5.169.

Pinch one nostril closed and ask the patient to breathe (Figure 5.170). Repeat the procedure and ask the patient which nostril he can breathe through better.

Select the most patent nostril (Figure 5.171).

Place the patient in a semi-upright position if his condition permits (Figure 5.172).

Slightly flex the head (Figure 5.173).

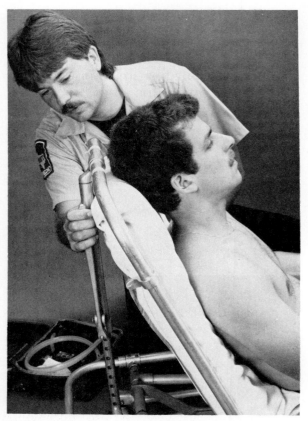

Figure 5.172.

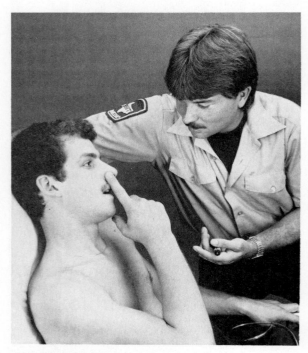

Figure 5.170.

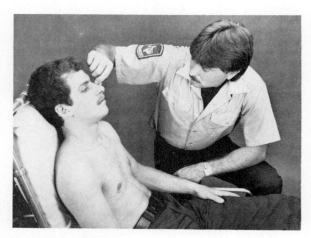

Figure 5.171.

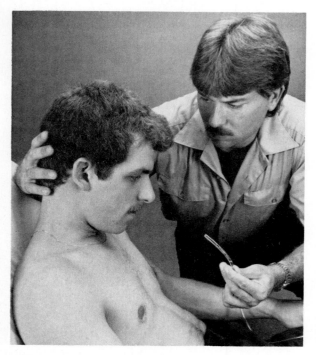

Figure 5.173.

Insert the lubricated tube into the most patent nostril (Figure 5.174).

Pass the tube carefully into the nose and along the nasal floor (Figure 5.175).

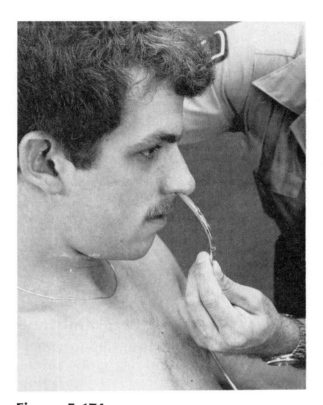

Figure 5.174.

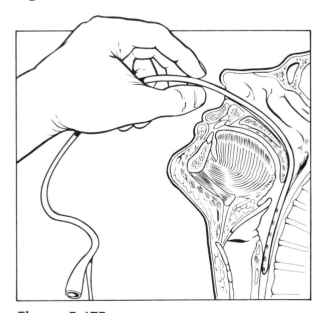

Figure 5.175.

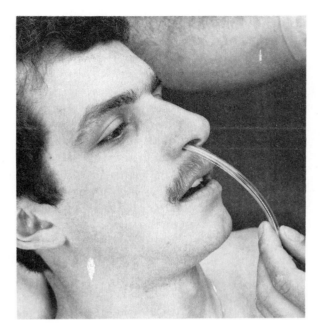

Figure 5.176.

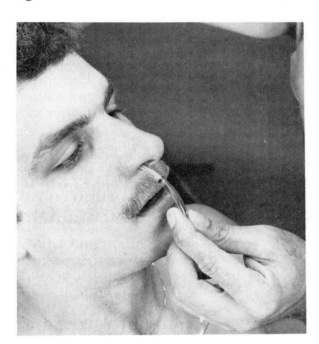

Figure 5.177.

Instruct the patient to swallow as the tube enters the oropharynx (Figure 5.176).

Pass the tube to the desired point as determined prior to intubation (Figure 5.177).

Check placement of the tube by aspirating gastric contents or by placing a stethoscope over the epigastrium and auscultating while injecting 20–30 mL of air into the tube (Figure 5.178).

Aspirate the stomach of its contents if indicated (Figure 5.179). Irrigation and aspiration should always occur concomitantly.

Irrigate if indicated (Figure 5.180).

Tape the tube in place and maintain suction if indicated (Figure 5.181).

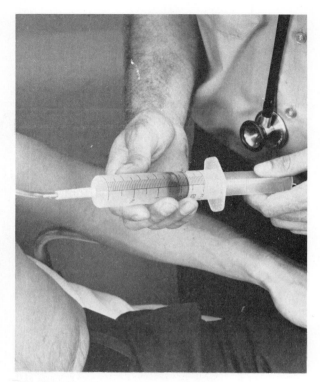

Figure 5.180.

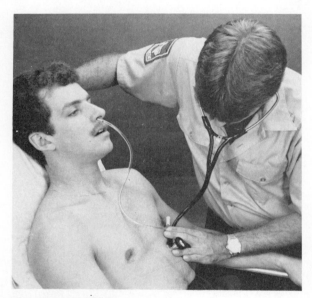

Figure 5.178.

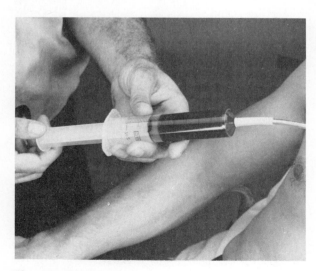

Figure 5.179.

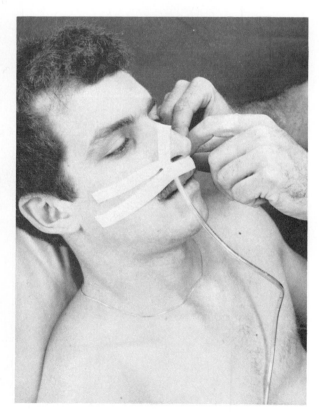

Figure 5.181.

STUDENT NAME ———————————————— **DATE** ——————

DIRECTIONS

Evaluate the student by using the criteria presented on this form. Mark PASS for an appropriate action. Mark FAIL for an inappropriate action or missed step. An asterisk (*) indicates an absolute step. Omission of this step indicates automatic failure.

STEP	PASS	FAIL
NASOGASTRIC TUBE INSERTION		
1. Receives the order	[ ]	[ ]
2. Prepares the equipment	[ ]	[ ]
3. Lubricates 6–8 inches of the distal part of the tube	[ ]	[ ]
4. Marks the distance the tube should be inserted	[ ]	[ ]
5. Examines the nose for septal deviation	[ ]	[ ]
6. Examines the nose for patency	[ ]	[ ]
7. Selects the most patent nostril	[ ]	[ ]
8. Places the patient in an upright, semi-sitting position	[ ]	[ ]
9. Explains the procedure to the patient*	[ ]	[ ]
10. Slightly flexes the head	[ ]	[ ]
11. Inserts the tube through the nose into the oropharynx	[ ]	[ ]
12. Instructs the patient to swallow as the tube enters the oropharynx	[ ]	[ ]
13. Passes the tube to the point determined earlier	[ ]	[ ]
14. Checks placement of the tube by aspirating gastric contents or by auscultation*	[ ]	[ ]
15. Tapes the tube in place	[ ]	[ ]

TOTAL SCORE (2 points for each PASS) ——————
(21 required for PASS)
NO ABSOLUTES MAY BE FAILED

——————————————————   ——————————————————
Evaluator   Date

Chapter Objectives

Upon completion of this chapter, the student should be able to:

1. List the indications, contraindications, precautions, and common complications of the following procedures:
   a. Monitoring of the EKG
   b. Defibrillation
   c. Cardioversion
   d. Carotid sinus massage

2. Be able to perform the following procedures according to the criteria presented:
   a. Monitoring of the EKG
   b. Defibrillation
   c. Cardioversion
   d. Carotid sinus massage

6

Cardiac-Related Skills

Monitoring of the EKG

Overview

The electrocardiogram (EKG) is a recording of the electrical activity of the heart and provides a great deal of information concerning the cardiac status of a patient. Because of this, the EKG is frequently monitored in both pre-hospital and inhospital care.

In routine medical practice a 12-lead EKG tracing is usually taken. However, for monitoring purposes, only one or two leads are generally used.

There are two methods of monitoring a patient's EKG. Static monitoring involves the actual recording of the patient's EKG onto graph paper. Dynamic monitoring, on the other hand, involves displaying the EKG on an oscilloscope. Both methods are used in prehospital care, and paramedics should be able to recognize dysrhythmias on either device.

Most EKG monitors used in prehospital care are combination EKG monitor/defibrillators (Figure 6.1). They are generally battery operated and are capable of dynamic monitoring or static recording of a patient's EKG.

Generally, leads I, II, or MCL1 (modified chest lead 1) are used. The monitoring device requires three leads: a positive lead, a negative lead, and a ground. Each of the common monitoring leads is simply a variation in the placement of the electrodes.

In the following description of lead placements it should be kept in mind that for general prehospital and inhospital monitoring the limb leads (for example, the left arm) are placed on the thorax at a point close to that limb.

In lead I the positive electrode is on the left arm, and the negative lead is on the right arm (Figure 6.2).

In lead II, the positive electrode is placed on the left leg, and the negative electrode is placed on the right arm (Figure 6.3). This lead is fairly popular because its position is quite similar to the normal electrical axis of the heart.

When using MCL1, the negative electrode is placed on the left shoulder, and the positive electrode is placed on the right leg (Figure 6.4). This lead is particularly useful when monitoring for the presence of ectopic beats.

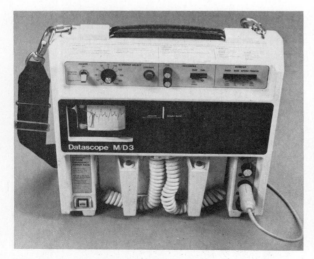

Figure 6.1. Typical EKG/Monitor defibrillator used in prehospital care.

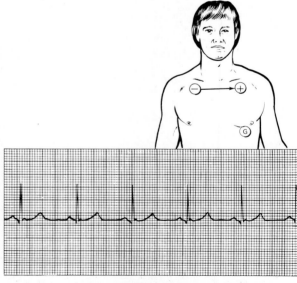

Figure 6.2. Electrode placement and typical lead I tracing.

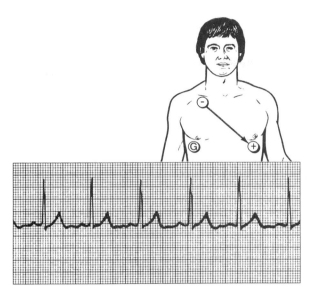

Figure 6.3. Electrode placement and typical lead II tracing.

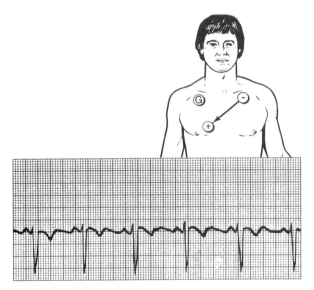

Figure 6.4. Electrode placement and typical MCL1 tracing.

Indications

EKG monitoring is indicated in any critical patient and in any patient where cardiac disease is thought to be present or any patient with an irregular pulse.

Contraindications

None.

Precautions

Some patients may become alarmed when you attempt to attach monitoring electrodes to them. Prior to placing the electrodes you should adequately explain to the patient what you are attempting to do. When placing electrodes on female patients you often must remove or pull up the blouse and any underwear which may be in the way. Again, it is important to explain to the patient what you are going to do and, at all times, keep the patient covered. When placing the modified left or right leg (lower) electrodes on a female patient's chest, it may be necessary to lift the breasts out of the way. Often the patient may prefer to do this for you.

It is often a difficult matter to attach electrodes to patients who are extremely diaphoretic. To help maintain attachment, benzoin spray may be applied to the skin prior to the electrodes.

Complications

Improper placement or loose electrodes may cause artifacts that may be mistaken for dysrhythmias.

Required Equipment

- EKG monitor
- Disposable electrodes
- Patient cable
- Benzoin spray

Procedure

Explain to the patient what you are going to do.

Turn on the monitor.

Remove or pull back clothing that may interfere with the procedure (Figure 6.7).

Prepare the patient cables (Figure 6.8).

Prepare the adhesive pads (Figure 6.9).

Apply the monitoring electrodes to obtain the desired lead (Figure 6.10).

Observe monitor (Figure 6.11).

Record tracing for the patient report (Figure 6.12).

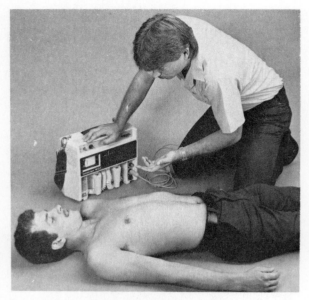

Figure 6.5. Explain to the patient what you are going to do.

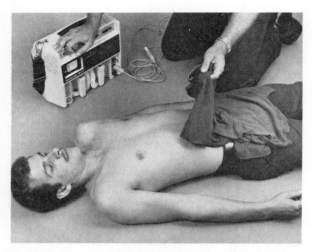

Figure 6.7. Remove or pull back any clothing that may interfere with the procedure.

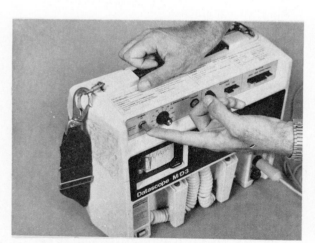

Figure 6.6. Turn on the monitor.

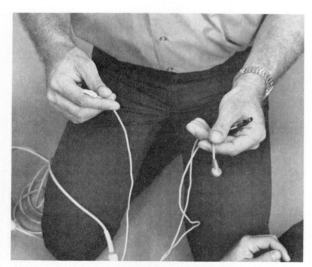

Figure 6.8. Prepare the patient cables.

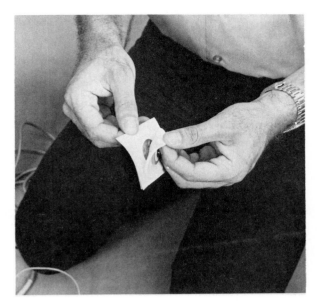

Figure 6.9. Prepare the adhesive pads.

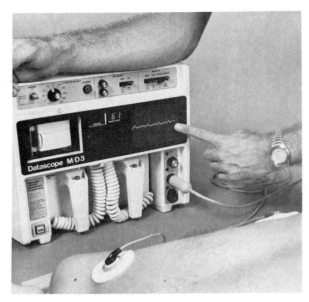

Figure 6.11. Observe monitor.

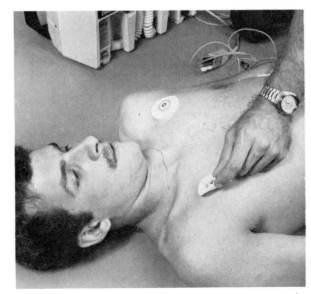

Figure 6.10. Apply the monitoring electrodes to obtain the desired lead.

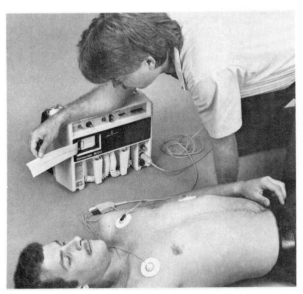

Figure 6.12. Record tracing for the patient report.

STUDENT NAME _____ **DATE** _____

DIRECTIONS

   Evaluate the student by using the criteria presented on this form. Mark PASS for an appropriate action. Mark FAIL for an inappropriate action or missed step. An asterisk (*) indicates an absolute step. Omission of this step indicates automatic failure.

STEP	PASS	FAIL
EKG MONITORING		
1. Explains procedure to the patient*	[ ]	[ ]
2. Turns on the monitor	[ ]	[ ]
3. Removes clothing that may be in the way	[ ]	[ ]
4. Prepares the patient cable	[ ]	[ ]
5. Prepares adhesive pads	[ ]	[ ]
6. Places electrodes in lead II position	[ ]	[ ]
7. Explains location of electrodes for lead I	[ ]	[ ]
8. Explains location of electrodes for MCL1	[ ]	[ ]
9. Observes monitor	[ ]	[ ]
10. Obtains rhythm strip	[ ]	[ ]

TOTAL SCORE (2 points for each PASS)   _____
(14 required for PASS)
NO ABSOLUTES MAY BE FAILED

_____   _____

                    Evaluator   Date

Static and Dynamic Dysrhythmia Recognition

Overview

This section is designed as a review of both standard and dynamic dys-rhythmias. The static tracings are actual EKGs taken from a patient suffering an acute myocardial infarction. It is, of course, impossible to actually present

Static Tracings

Identify the dysrhythmia illustrated in the static EKG tracings in Figures 6.13–6.32.

Interpretation of Dysrhythmias

Static

6.13 Sinus arrhythmia
6.14 Ventricular fibrillation
6.15 Atrial flutter

6.16 Third degree heart block
6.17 Ventricular tachycardia
6.18 Sinus bradycardia
6.19 Second degree heart block (Mobitz II)
6.20 Normal sinus rhythm with PVCs (premature ventricular contraction)
6.21 Second degree heart block (Mobitz I) [Wenckebach]
6.22 Sinus bradycardia
6.23 Idioventricular rhythm
6.24 First degree heart block
6.25 Sinus tachycardia
6.26 Wandering atrial pacemaker
6.27 Asystole
6.28 Atrial fibrillation
6.29 Normal sinus rhythm with bigeminal PVCs
6.30 Junctional rhythm
6.31 Sinus arrest
6.32 Sinus tachycardia with PACs

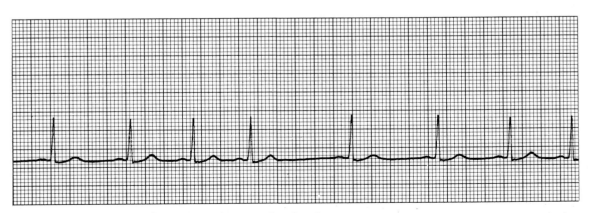

Figure 6.13. Dysrhythmia: _____

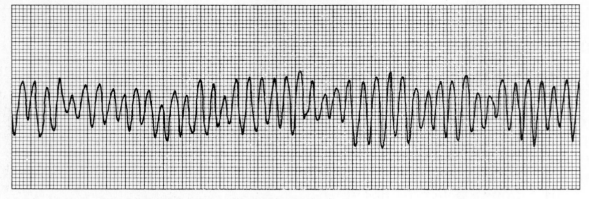

Figure 6.14. Dysrhythmia: _____

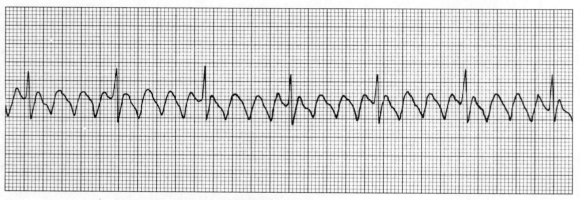

Figure 6.15. Dysrhythmia: _____

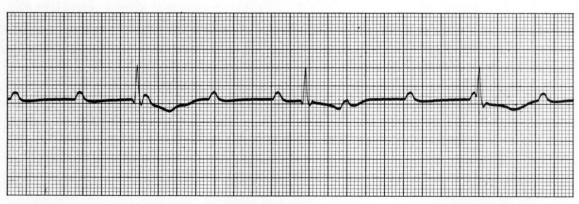

Figure 6.16. Dysrhythmia: _____

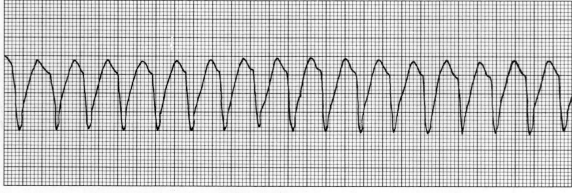

Figure 6.17. Dysrhythmia: _____

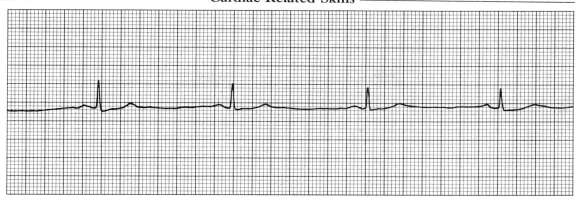

Figure 6.18. Dysrhythmia: _____

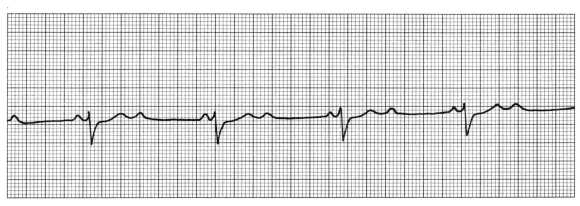

Figure 6.19. Dysrhythmia: _____

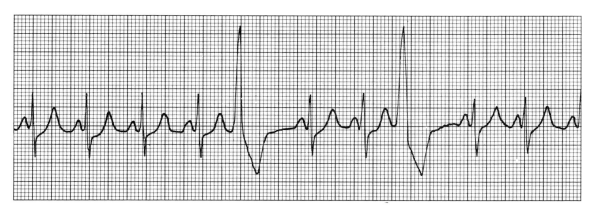

Figure 6.20. Dysrhythmia: _____

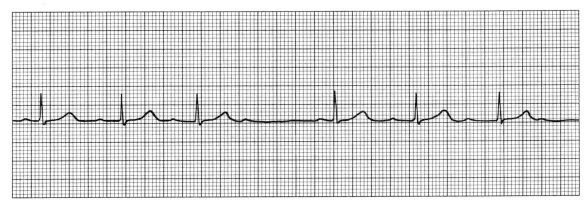

Figure 6.21. Dysrhythmia: _____

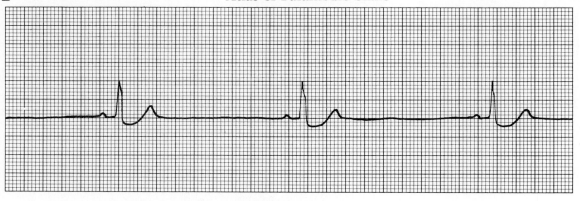

Figure 6.22. Dysrhythmia: _____

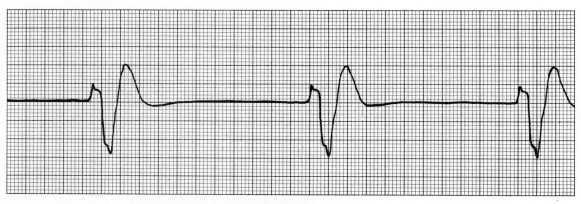

Figure 6.23. Dysrhythmia: _____

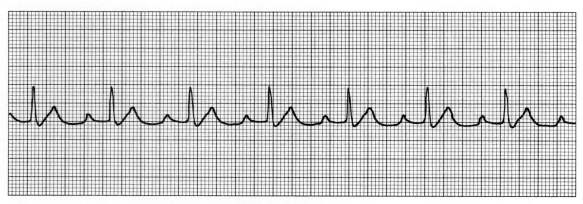

Figure 6.24. Dysrhythmia: _____

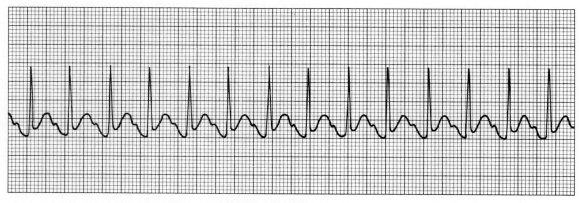

Figure 6.25. Dysrhythmia: _____

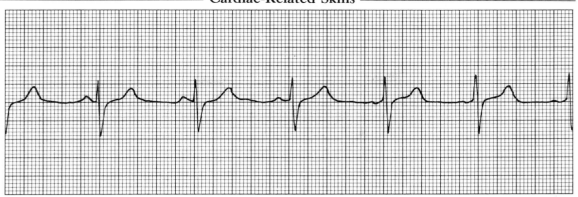

Figure 6.26. Dysrhythmia: _____

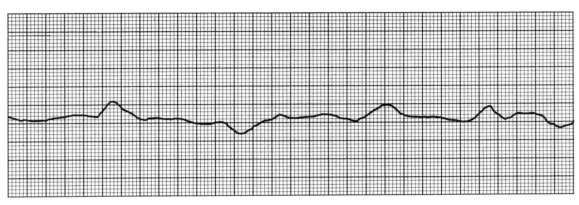

Figure 6.27. Dysrhythmia: _____

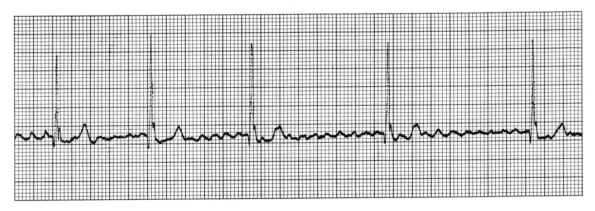

Figure 6.28. Dysrhythmia: _____

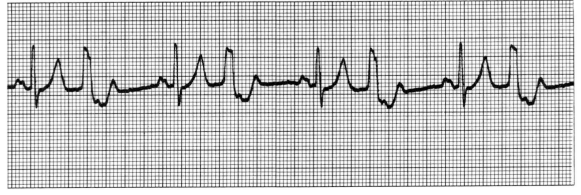

Figure 6.29. Dysrhythmia: _____

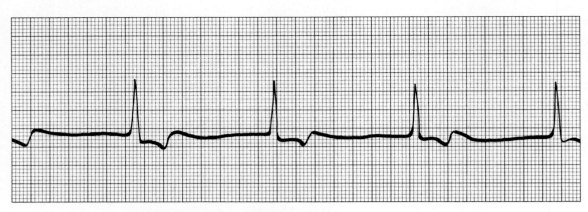

Figure 6.30. Dysrhythmia: _____

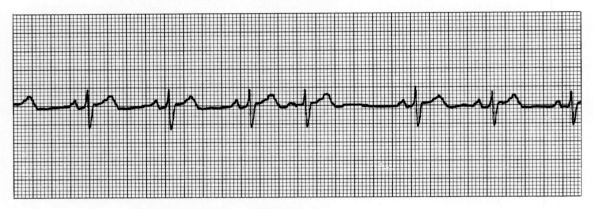

Figure 6.31. Dysrhythmia: _____

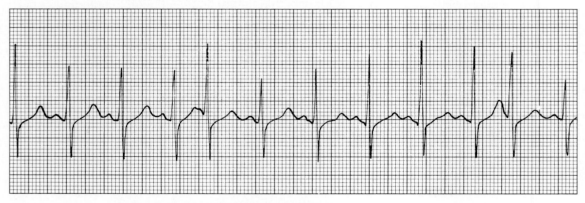

Figure 6.32. Dysrhythmia: _____

STUDENT NAME _____ **DATE** _____

DIRECTIONS

Evalute the student by using the criteria presented on this form. Mark PASS for an appropriate action. Mark FAIL for an inappropriate or missed step. An asterisk (*) indicates an absolute step. Omission of this step inidcates automatic failure.

THE STUDENT SHOULD BE ABLE TO IDENTIFY A STATIC ARRHYTHMIA WITHIN A 15-SECOND TIME LIMIT.

STEP	PASS	FAIL
STATIC ARRHYTHMIA		
6.13.	[ ]	[ ]
6.14.	[ ]	[ ]
6.15.	[ ]	[ ]
6.16.	[ ]	[ ]
6.17.	[ ]	[ ]
6.18.	[ ]	[ ]
6.19.	[ ]	[ ]
6.20.	[ ]	[ ]
6.21.	[ ]	[ ]
6.22.	[ ]	[ ]
6.23.	[ ]	[ ]
6.24.	[ ]	[ ]
6.25.	[ ]	[ ]
6.26.	[ ]	[ ]
6.27.	[ ]	[ ]
6.28.	[ ]	[ ]
6.29.	[ ]	[ ]
6.30.	[ ]	[ ]
6.31.	[ ]	[ ]
6.32.	[ ]	[ ]

TOTAL SCORE (2 points for each PASS) _____
(28 required for PASS)

_____ _____
Evaluator   Date

Electrical Defibrillation

Overview

Electrical defibrillation is the process of applying an electrical current to the myocardium in an effort to terminate an ineffective dysrhythmia such as ventricular fibrillation. Electrical defibrillation is effective in the management of ventricular fibrillation and nonperfusing ventricular tachycardia. In ventricular fibrillation the dominant pacemaker of the heart is lost. Many ectopic cells begin to fire randomly thus resulting in an ineffective rhythm that is incapable of pumping blood. Electrical defibrillation, properly applied, causes a complete depolarization of the entire myocardium. Following defibrillation, if physiological conditions are right, a dominant pacemaker will again fire and an organized rhythm can be restored.

An electrical defibrillator is a device capable of storing and delivering electrical energy to a patient by way of paddle electrodes. Most defibrillators available today are of the direct current (DC) variety and derive their energy from an internal battery source. When charged, the energy in the battery is transferred to a storage capacitor. Upon discharge, the capacitor delivers the stored energy to the patient. The strength of the defibrillation countershock, measured in joules (J), can be varied depending on the size of the patient. The unit joules, formerly called watt-seconds, is represented by the following equation:

$$\text{Energy} = \text{Power} \times \text{Duration}$$
$$\text{(joules)} \quad \text{(watts)} \quad \text{(seconds)}$$

The electrical defibrillator is a dangerous device that should only be used following proper training.

Indications

Electrical defibrillation is indicated in the management of ventricular fibrilla-tion and certain cases of nonperfusing ventricular tachycardia.

Contraindications

Electrical defibrillation is not indicated in any situation other than just described. Synchronized cardioversion, as opposed to defibrillation, is indicated in cases of paroxysmal supraventricular tachycardia and other perfusing dysrhythmias that require electrical intervention.

Precautions

When treating a suspected case of ventricular fibrillation, the patient's pulse must be continually monitored. Many factors, such as patient movement or loose electrodes, can mimic ventricular fibrillation.

Conductive electrical paste or pads should be applied prior to electrical defibrillation. Conductive paste reduces the electrical resistance between the paddles and the patient which results in a more effective transmission of energy and a reduction in the likelihood of causing electrical burns to the patient. Saline pads may be used when conductive paste is not available. However, in no instance should flammable liquids, such as isopropyl alcohol, be used.

Electrical defibrillation should not be attempted in environments where flammable gases are present. In these cases, the patient should be moved a safe distance from the hazardous environment before defibrillation is attempted.

It is also important to assure that the patient is not carrying, or in contact with, a loaded gun.

Defibrillators should only be tested according to the manufacturer's written instructions. Do not hold the paddles together and discharge the device unless the procedure is recommended by the manufacturer.

Prior to defibrillation, the synchronizer switch **must** be turned off.

Failure to do so will result in a delay in delivering the charge to the patient as the synchronizer will prevent the device from discharging because of the absence of a QRS complex as seen in ventricular fibrillation.

IT IS ESSENTIAL THAT NO ONE BE IN CONTACT WITH THE PATIENT OR THE DEFIBRILLATOR AT THE TIME OF DISCHARGE. IMMEDIATELY PRIOR TO DISCHARGE THE OPERATOR SHOULD SHOUT A WARNING SUCH AS "CLEAR" OR "STAND BACK" BEFORE DISCHARGING THE DEVICE.

Complications

Complications associated with electrical defibrillation include arcing of the charge between the two paddles, burning of the patient's chest, myocardial damage, and possible injury to the operator.

Required Equipment

- DC Defibrillator (Figure 6.33)
- Electrode paste
- Defibrillator batteries

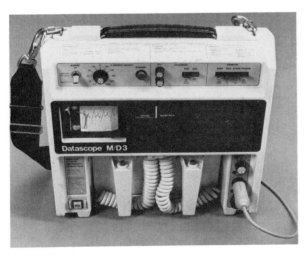

Figure 6.33. Typical battery-powered defibrillator.

Procedure

Confirm that the patient is apneic by standard BLS technique (Figure 6.34).

Confirm pulselessness by palpating for a carotid pulse (Figure 6.35). Start CPR.

Turn on the defibrillator/monitor (Figure 6.36).

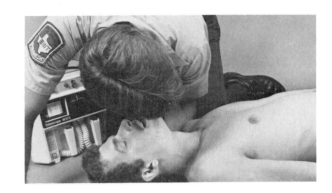

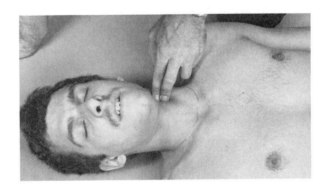

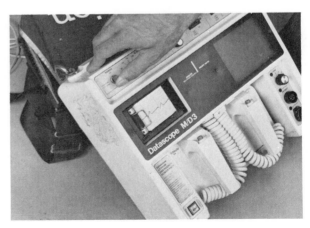

Figure 6.36.

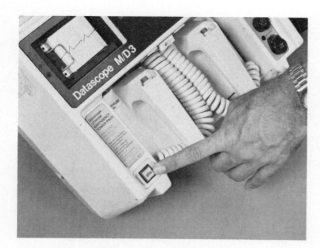

Figure 6.37.

Make sure the synchronizer switch is off (Figure 6.37).

Apply electrode paste to the paddles (Figure 6.38).

Place the quick-look paddles on the patient's chest (Figure 6.39).

Properly place the paddles (Figure 6.40).

Confirm ventricular fibrillation (Figure 6.41).

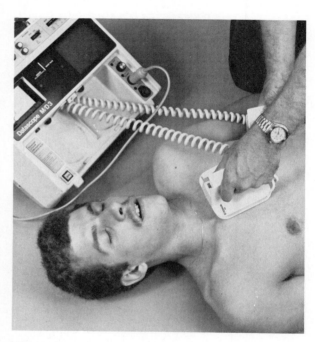

Figure 6.39.

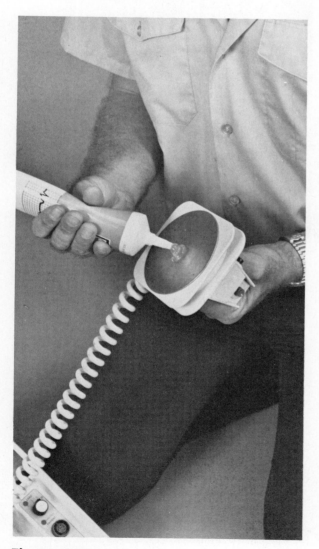

Figure 6.38.

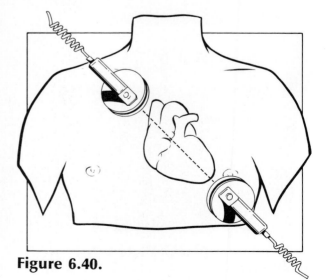

Figure 6.40.

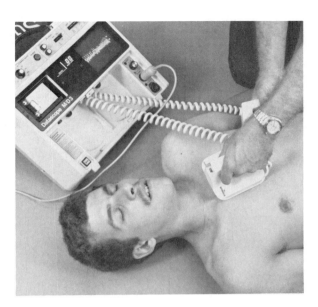

Figure 6.41.

Charge the defibrillator to the desired setting (Figure 6.42).

Check to make sure that no one is in contact with the patient. Shout "Clear" (Figure 6.43).

Apply approximately 10 kg (25 lb) of pressure and discharge the paddles (Figure 6.44).

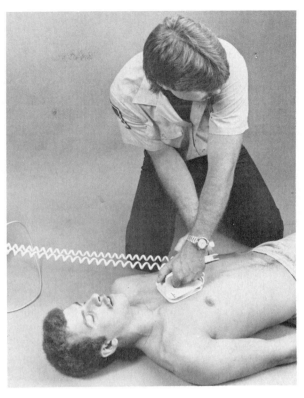

Figure 6.43.

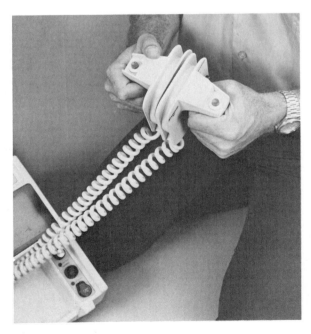

Figure 6.42.

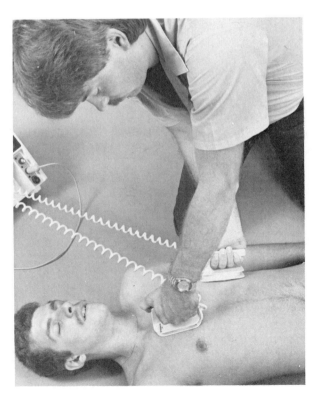

Figure 6.44.

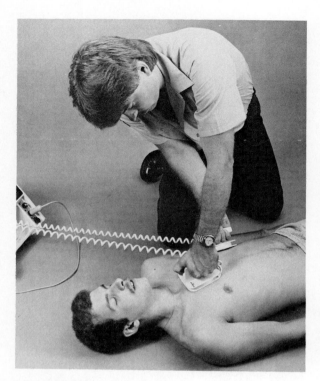

Figure 6.45.

Maintain quick-look paddles in contact with the patient and monitor the rhythm or place standard monitoring leads on the patient (Figure 6.45).

Recheck the pulse (Figure 6.46).

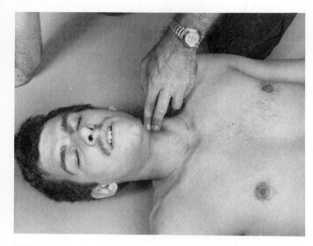

Figure 6.46.

STUDENT NAME _____ **DATE** _____

DIRECTIONS

Evalute the student by using the criteria presented on this form. Mark PASS for an appropriate action. Mark FAIL for an inappropriate or missed step. An asterisk (*) indicates an absolute step. Omission of this step inidcates automatic failure.

STEP		PASS	FAIL
1.	Confirms apnea*	[ ]	[ ]
2.	Confirms pulselessness*	[ ]	[ ]
3.	Turns on the defibrillator/monitor	[ ]	[ ]
4.	Assures that the synchronizer switch is in the off position*	[ ]	[ ]
5.	Applies electrode paste to the paddles	[ ]	[ ]
6.	Places quick-look paddles on the patient's chest	[ ]	[ ]
7.	Confirms ventricular fibrillation*	[ ]	[ ]
8.	Charges the defibrillator to the appropriate setting	[ ]	[ ]
9.	Checks to assure that no one is in contact with the patient or the defibrillator*	[ ]	[ ]
10.	Shouts "Clear"*	[ ]	[ ]
11.	Discharges paddles	[ ]	[ ]
12.	Maintains paddle position on the patient's chest to monitor rhythm	[ ]	[ ]
13.	Checks pulse	[ ]	[ ]
14.	Prepares for ACLS	[ ]	[ ]

TOTAL SCORE (2 points for each PASS) _____
(20 required for PASS)
NO ABSOLUTES MAY BE FAILED

_____   _____
Evaluator   Date

Synchronized Cardioversion

Overview

Synchronized cardioversion is the application of an electrical countershock to a patient during a specific part of the cardiac cycle. It has proven effective in the treatment of highly symptomatic tachydysrhythmias such as paroxysmal supraventricular tachycardia and atrial fibrillation which fail to respond to other definitive treatment modalities. Synchronized cardioversion is only possible with DC defibrillators that are equipped with a synchronizer. The synchronizer is able to recognize and mark the R wave of the QRS complex (Figure 6.47). When the discharge button is pressed, the synchronizer will only allow the countershock to be delivered on the R wave, thus avoiding the vulnerable period associated with the T wave. This avoidance significantly reduced the likelihood of inducing ventricular fibrillation. Furthermore, less energy is required because the countershock is delivered at a specific point during the cardiac cycle.

Indications

Synchronized cardioversion is indicated for the treatment of supraventricular, and occasionally ventricular, dysrhythmias in clinical settings (such as severe hypotension) that require rapid dysrhythmia termination to prevent further deterioration of the patient.

Contraindications

Synchronized cardioversion is not indicated in the prehospital setting in any situation other than that just described. Electrical defibrillation is indicated in cases of ventricular fibrillation and nonperfusing ventricular tachycardia.

Precautions

The same precautions apply to synchronized cardioversion as apply to electrical defibrillation. In addition, it is important to remember that most synchronizers are designed to recognize an R wave that is positively deflected. In cases where the electrical axis of the patient is deviated to a point where the R wave is negatively deflected, it may be necessary to change the monitoring leads before the machine will mark the R wave.

Cases may occur where you will be called upon to deliver a synchronized countershock to a rapidly deteriorating patient who is still conscious. Because the procedure is less than pleasant, you may want to premedicate the patient with intravenous diazepan (Valium®), if time permits, before applying the countershock. This will induce drowsiness and will often reduce the patient's recall of the procedure.

Complications

The same complications apply to synchronized cardioversion as apply to electrical defibrillation. It is important to

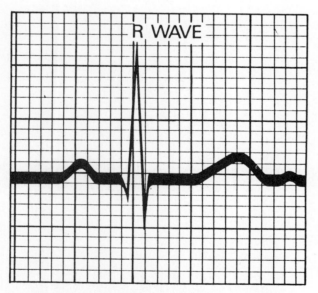

Figure 6.47. R Wave of the QRS complex.

remember that synchronized cardioversion can occasionally induce ventricular fibrillation. If this occurs, immediately turn off the synchronizer switch and defibrilate the patient in the manner described in the previous section.

Required Equipment

- DC Defibrillator with synchronizer
- Electrode paste
- 10 mg of injectible diazepan (Valium)

Procedure

Receive orders from the base-section physician (Figure 6.48).

Confirm the presence of the dysrhythmia and the clinical status of the patient (Figure 6.49).

If required, premedicate the patient (Figure 6.50).

Turn on the defibrillator and the synchronizer switch (Figure 6.51).

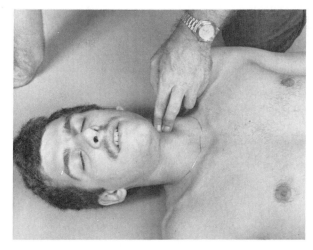

Figure 6.49.

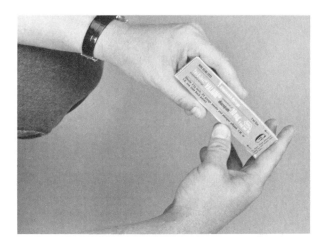

Figure 6.50.

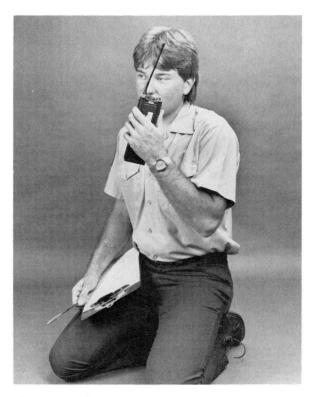

Figure 6.48.

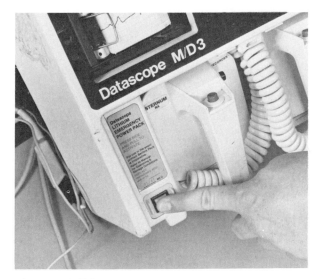

Figure 6.51.

Apply electrode paste to the paddles (Figure 6.52).

Charge the paddles to the desired setting (Figure 6.53). Assure that the synchronizer is still on and is still marking the R wave.

Press and HOLD the discharge but-tons until the countershock is delivered (Figure 6.54).

CHECK THE PULSE and the monitor for any change (Figure 6.55).

Confirm delivery of the countershock and the results to the base-station physician (Figure 6.56).

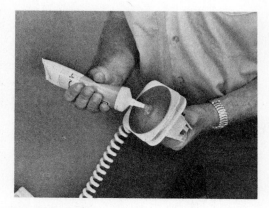

Figure 6.52.

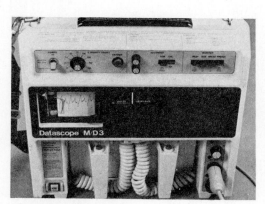

Figure 6.53.

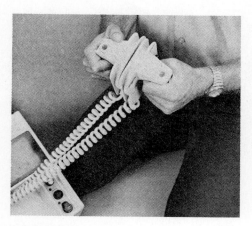

Figure 6.54.

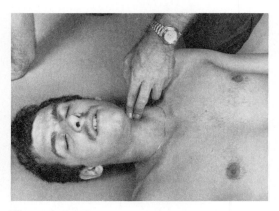

Figure 6.55.

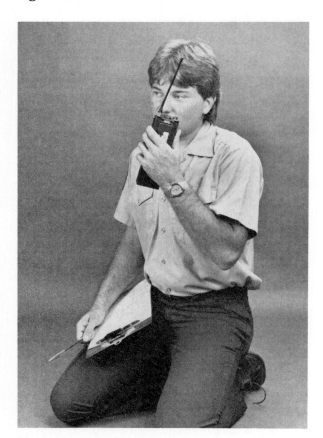

Figure 6.56.

STUDENT NAME _____ **DATE** _____

DIRECTIONS

Evalute the student by using the criteria presented on this form. Mark PASS for an appropriate action. Mark FAIL for an inappropriate or missed step. An asterisk (*) indicates an absolute step. Omission of this step inidcates automatic failure.

STEP	PASS	FAIL
1. Receives order*	[ ]	[ ]
2. Confirms the dysrhythmia	[ ]	[ ]
3. If required, premedicates the patient	[ ]	[ ]
4. Turns on the defibrillator/monitor	[ ]	[ ]
5. Assures that the synchronizer switch is in the on position*	[ ]	[ ]
6. Assures that the synchronizer is marking the R wave*	[ ]	[ ]
7. Applies electrode paste to the paddles	[ ]	[ ]
8. Charges the paddles to the appropriate setting	[ ]	[ ]
9. Checks to assure that no one is in contact with the patient or the defibrillator*	[ ]	[ ]
10. Shouts "Clear"*	[ ]	[ ]
11. Presses and HOLDS discharge buttons	[ ]	[ ]
12. Checks the pulse and the monitor	[ ]	[ ]
13. Prepares to immediately defibrillate if ventricular fibrillation is accidentally induced*	[ ]	[ ]
14. Confirms delivery of the countershock with the base-station physician	[ ]	[ ]

TOTAL SCORE (2 points for each PASS)   _____
(20 required for PASS)
NO ABSOLUTES MAY BE FAILED

_____   _____
                Evaluator   Date

Carotid Sinus Massage

Overview

Carotid sinus massage is an effective method of stimulating the vagus nerve (Figure 6.57) and is often effective in slowing tachydysrhythmias such as paroxysmal supraventricular tachycardia. The vagus nerve is the tenth cranial nerve and carries parasympathetic nerve fibers to the heart and other organs. Stimulation of the vagus nerve causes a slowing of the heart rate. The vagus nerve exits the brain and passes through the neck in close association with the carotid artery. The nerve can often be stimulated manually by applying firm, steady pressure on the carotid artery near the angle of the jaw.

Other methods of stimulating the vagus nerve include having the patient hold his breath or bearing down as if moving his bowels (Valsalva maneuver).

Indications

Carotid sinus massage is indicated in the treatment of paroxysmal supraventricular tachycardia (formerly PAT) that is symptomatic.

Contraindications

Carotid sinus massage should not be attempted in patients who have a history of stroke (CVA) or known disease of the carotid arteries. It is always a good practice, especially in elderly individuals, to auscultate for bruits as described in Chapter 1.

Precautions

Occasionally, in susceptible individuals, carotid sinus massage may result in asystole or ventricular fibrillation. Because of this, all patients receiving carotid sinus massage should be on the monitor and an intravenous infusion of 5% dextrose in water should be initiated. Emergency medications and ACLS

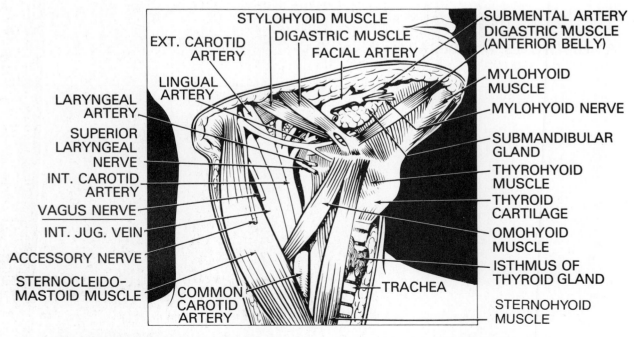

Figure 6.57. Anatomy of the vagus nerve as it passes through the neck.

equipment should be immediately available.

NEVER massage both carotid arteries at the same time.

Complications

Bradydysrhythmias sometimes occur following carotid sinus massage. These may result in hypotension or unconsciousness. In addition, as mentioned previously, asystole may occur in susceptible individuals.

Required Equipment

- EKG Monitor
- IV 5% dextrose
- ACLS equipment

Procedure

Receive the order from the base-station physician (Figure 6.58).

Assure that an IV is initiated and the patient is being monitored (Figure 6.59).

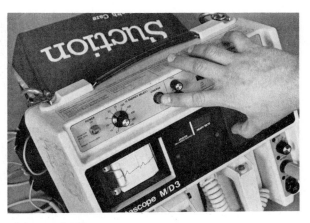

Figure 6.59.

Assure that ACLs equipment is ready (Figure 6.60).

Gently palpate both carotid arteries SEPARATELY to assure that there are equal pulses (Figure 6.61). If a pulse is absent or weak on one side, the procedure should not be carried out. Auscultate for bruits.

Locate the carotid sinus on the right side of the neck (Figure 6.62). This sinus is anterior to the sternocleidomastoid muscle near the angle of the jaw.

Turn the patient's head slightly to the left side (Figure 6.63).

With two fingers, firmly press the carotid artery against the transverse process of the cervical vertebra (Figure 6.64). You should be able to feel the

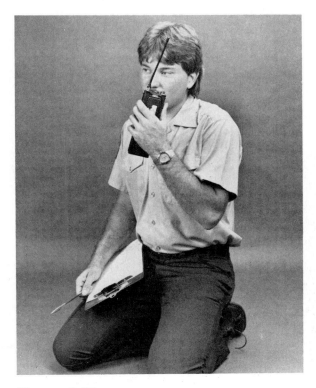

Figure 6.58.

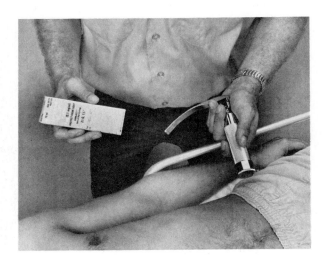

Figure 6.60.

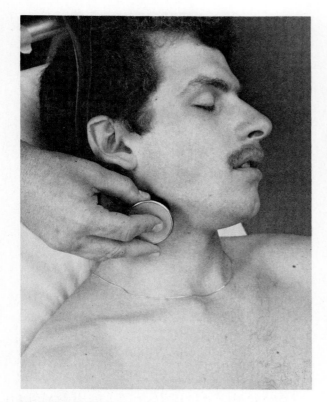

Figure 6.61.

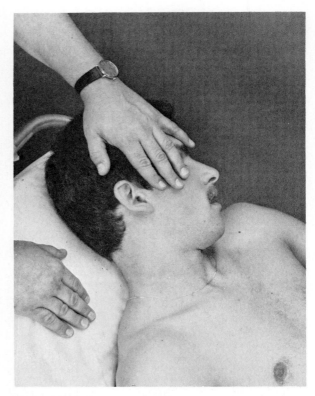

Figure 6.63.

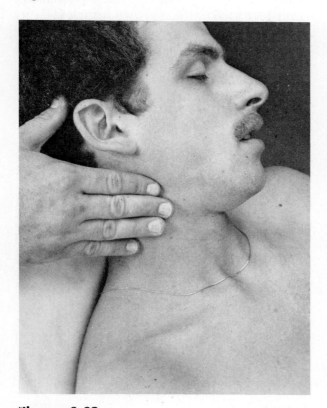

Figure 6.62.

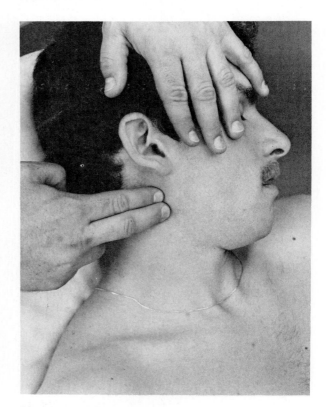

Figure 6.64.

pulse below your fingertips. Press for no longer than 15–20 seconds while simultaneously massaging the area with your fingers. KEEP AN EYE ON THE MONITOR AT ALL TIMES. Stop immediately if the rate begins to slow.

If massage of the right carotid is unsuccessful, then wait 2–3 minutes and repeat the procedure on the left side (Figure 6.65).

Report the results of the procedure to the base-station physician (Figure 6.66).

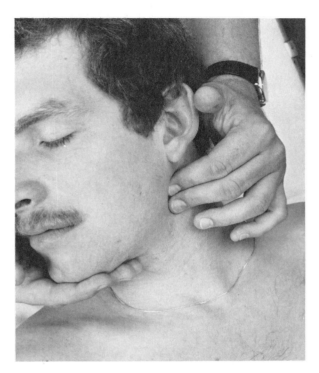

Figure 6.65.

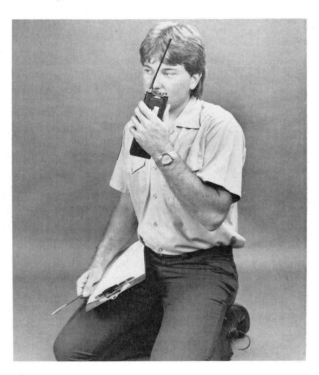

Figure 6.66.

STUDENT NAME _____ **DATE** _____

DIRECTIONS

Evalute the student by using the criteria presented on this form. Mark PASS for an appropriate action. Mark FAIL for an inappropriate or missed step. An asterisk (*) indicates an absolute step. Omission of this step inidcates automatic failure.

STEP	PASS	FAIL
Carotid Sinus Massage		
1. Receives order*	[ ]	[ ]
2. Understands indications and contraindications*	[ ]	[ ]
3. Assures that an IV is established*	[ ]	[ ]
4. Assures that ACLS equipment is nearby*	[ ]	[ ]
5. Checks to make sure monitor is on*	[ ]	[ ]
6. Palpates both carotids separately to assure that there are equal pulses	[ ]	[ ]
7. Locates the carotid sinus on the right side of the neck	[ ]	[ ]
8. Turns the patient's head slightly to the left side	[ ]	[ ]
9. Massages the right carotid sinus for no longer than 15–20 seconds	[ ]	[ ]
10. If unsuccessful, waits 2–3 minutes before attempting other side*	[ ]	[ ]

TOTAL SCORE (2 points for each PASS) _____
(14 required for PASS)
NO ABSOLUTES MAY BE FAILED

_____   _____
                Evaluator   Date

Chapter Objectives

Upon completion of this chapter, the student should be able to:

1. Prepare and present a complete and accurate oral patient report over a radio following accepted local protocols.
2. Prepare a complete written patient report by using the SOAP format or another format as approved by the regional medical director.
3. Understand the need for an accurate and legible patient report.

7

Communications Skills

The paramedic and EMT-intermediate must be capable of communicating information concerning a patient both verbally and in writing. In the field, the paramedic must function as the eyes, ears, and hands of a remote base-station physician. To do this effectively, the paramedic must be able to organize the information gained from the patient assessment into a logical format for presentation to the base-station physician. Following the emergency response, an adequate and detailed patient report must be prepared with much of the same information presented in the verbal radio report.

This chapter will present a discussion of both the verbal patient report and the written run report.

Reporting of Patient Information over the Radio

Although the format for presenting a patient report varies from system to sytem, most systems are similar to the format used in performing the patient assessment, namely the SOAP format. The following format is commonly employed in EMS. (An example is shown in Example 1.)

1. Establish communications.
2. Identify your unit and yourself.
3. Assure that the base station is receiving you properly.
4. Present the following information:
   a. age and sex of the patient and mental status
   b. chief complaint
   c. general condition of the patient (amount of distress)
   d. background of the chief complaint
   e. pertinent parts of medical history
   f. current medications
   g. allergies
   h. objective findings
      1. vital signs
      2. pertinent aspects of the physical exam
      3. transmit EKG if requested
   i. treatment plan
   j. proposed destination
5. Physician direction
6. Confirmation of orders
7. Patient response to treatment
8. Termination of the report

The example is clear and to the point. Nonessential information is omitted. The paramedic and the physician collaborated regarding the treatment plan and interpretation of the EKG. This collaboration is essential for good and efficient patient care.

The Written Report

The written report, generally completed following delivery of the patient to the hospital, is essential. The written report is the permanent medical record for the patient and should include such things as name, date, pertinent data, signs and symptoms, response times, patient care data, assessment, intervention, and disposition. The patient report serves to protect both the patient and the paramedic.

It is best to present the medical information concerning the patient in the SOAP format. Unusual terminology and abbreviations should not be used. The examples shown in Figures 7.1–7.6 are patient report forms from different parts of the country that have been completed appropriately.

Example 1.

Speaker	Transmission
Paramedic:	"706 to Biotel."
Base Station:	"This is Biotel, go ahead 706."
Paramedic:	"I need a doctor in medicine."
Base Station:	"Standby 706."
Doctor:	"This is Dr. Gallagher, go ahead 706."
Paramedic:	"We have been called to the scene of a 59-year-old male patient who is alert and complaining of severe, crushing substernal chest pain. The patient is in moderate to severe distress. The pain began approximately one hour ago, shortly after he arrived home from work. He has a history of heart disease and hypertension and is a current patient of Dr. Goldblatt. He is currently taking nitroglycerin, Lanoxin, Lasix, and Inderal. He states that he is allergic to sulfa drugs. His vital signs are as follows: blood pressure of 140/100/80, pulse of 110 and regular, and respirations of 24, rapid and labored. He is pale and diaphoretic. There is a moderate amount of jugular venous distension. There also appears to be some pedal edema. Stand by for EKG telemetry."
Doctor:	"I read sinus tachycardia"
Paramedic:	"We read the same. We would like permission to administer oxygen at 6 L/min via mask, start an IV of 5% dextrose in water, and transport to Baylor."
Doctor:	"O.K., go ahead and administer oxygen at 6 L/min and start an IV of 5% dextrose in water. Did you say he was allergic to any medicines?"
Paramedic:	"That's affirmative, he is allergic to sulfa drugs."
Doctor:	"Is his pain still severe?"
Paramedic:	"That's affirmative, Biotel."
Doctor:	"After you get the IV started, administer 1 nitroglycerin tablet. If that doesn't relieve the pain, then administer 4 mg of morphine sulfate IV."
Paramedic:	"Received, confirming an order for oxygen at 6 L/min, an IV of 5% dextrose in water, 1 nitroglycerin tablet sublingually, and if the pain is not relieved, 4 mg of morphine IV."
Doctor:	"That's correct."
Paramedic:	"Are we clear to Baylor?"
Doctor:	"That's affirmative, proceed to Baylor ER. We will advise them of this patient."
Paramedic:	"Received, 706 clear."
Base Station:	"706 Clear."

DALLAS FIRE DEPARTMENT
EMERGENCY MEDICAL SERVICES

PATIENT FORM

FALSE OR
NO TRANSPORT 1 2 3 4 5 6

☑ Dry ☐ Rain ☐ Snow ☐ Ice ☐ Fog
WEATHER CONDITIONS

86-201
INCIDENT NUMBER

_1_ OF _1_
PATIENTS

Police # ____ ☑ On Scene ☐ Requested

Date _2/15/86_ Time _1530_ Charge ____

Doctor's Name ____ ☐ On Scene ☐ Requested

Location _1601 S. HARWOOD_ Hospital _PARKLAND_

Patient Name _JASON SMITH_ Birthdate _2/21/42_ M ✓ / F Race _W_ Wt _215_

Patient # Assigned at Hosp If Known _47326-41_

Street _5601 Allison_ City & State _DALLAS, TX_ Zip _75021_

Responsible Adult _SAM?_ Relationship ____ Phone ____

Drivers License # _0743262 - TX_ Medicare # ____ Medicaid # ____

Employer _City of DALLAS_ Soc. Sec. # ____

Paramedic _JOHNSON_ No. _431_ MICU # _704_ Shift _C_

Paramedic/Driver _DeLOACH_ No. _1602_ Responded From _STATION 4_

Vital Signs: B P _110/60_ Pulse _84_ Resp. _22_ Allergies _NKA_

Left margin vertical text: WHITE — Hospital, YELLOW — Tax, PINK — File, GOLD — Paramedic

SEVERITY	TYPE OF INJURY OR ILLNESS		DRUGS	AID PROVIDED BY PARAMEDIC/EMT
Consciousness (Con) Semi Unc	1 ☐ Agg. Assault 2 ☑ Alcohol 3 ☐ Asthma 4 ☑ Auto Accident 5 ☐ Bite/Sting 6 ☐ Burn 7 ☐ Convulsions 8 ☑ Cuts/Bruises 9 ☐ Diabetic 10 ☐ Drowning 11 ☐ Drug Reaction 12 ☐ Dyspnea 13 ☐ Electrocution 14 ☐ Emer. Trans. 15 ☐ Emphysema 16 ☐ Fainted 17 ☐ Female Comp. 18 ☐ Flu 19 ☑ Fracture 20 ☐ GI Complaint 21 ☐ Gunshot 22 ☐ Heart 23 ☐ Hypervent. 24 ☐ Hypoglycemia 25 ☐ Maternity	26 ☐ Medical Emer. 27 ☐ Muscle/Skeletal 28 ☐ Overdose 29 ☐ Poisoning 30 ☐ Psychiatric 31 ☐ Shock 32 ☐ Sickle Cell 33 ☐ Stabbing 34 ☐ Stroke 35 ☐ Suffocation 36 ☐ Suicide 37 ☐ T.B. 38 ☐ VD 39 ☐ None 40 ☐ Other (Specify) **RESPONSE CODE TO HOSPITAL** ☑ 1 ☐ 3	A ☐ Sodium Bicarb B ☐ Lidocaine 1% C ☐ Lidocaine 4% D ☐ Atropine E ☐ Isuprel F ☐ Levophed G ☐ Epinephrine H ☐ Calcium Chl. I ☐ Benadryl J ☐ Valium K ☐ Dextrose 50% L ☐ Nitronox M ☐ Narcan N ☐ Alcaine O ☐ Ipecac P ☐ Burn Spray Q ☐ Epine. 1:1000 R ☐ Lasix S ☐ Bretylol **IV** 1 ☑ Ringers Lac. 2 ☐ D5W	A ☐ EKG B ☐ Telemetry C ☑ IV D ☐ Drugs E ☐ Defib-Suc. F ☐ Defib-Unsuc. G ☐ Esoph-Airway H ☐ Intubated I ☑ Oxygen J ☐ CPR-Suc. K ☐ CPR-Unsuc. L ☐ Cont. Bleed M ☑ Bandaging N ☑ Splinting O ☐ Spine Board P ☐ Anti-Shock Q ☐ OB-Live Br. R ☐ OB-Still Br. S ☐ Rotating TK T ☐ Trans. Only U ☐ None V ☐ Other W ☐ CPR Citizen X ☐ CPR Thumper Y ☐ MAST Trousers Z ☐ Dextrostix
Bleeding Non Min (Mod) Sev				
Pain Non (Min) Mod Sev				
☐ DOS ☐ DOA				
LOCATION OF INJURY-ILLNESS ☑ Head ☐ Face ☐ Eye L/R ☐ Neck ☑ Back ☑ Chest ☐ Abdomen ☐ Pelvic Region ☑ Upper Extremity (L)/R ☐ Lower Extremity L/R ☐ Respiratory ☐ Cardiovascular ☐ Other				

Chief Complaint _Multiple cuts & fractures 2° TO MVA_

Remarks _Pt. involved in 2 car MVA. Driver of car struck on (L). Trapped for 15 minutes._

Aid Provided By

Fire Co. # _3_

Other ____

If Interhospital Transfer, ER Doctor authorizing move: ____

I was offered aid by the City of Dallas Emergency Medical Service. I chose not to accept Emergency Treatment and/or Transportation

Signature ____ Witness ____

Doctor or R.N. signature below does not approve or disapprove above information

DFD Form 200 Revised SEP 80   FRD-00981

Dr. or R.N. _____
SIGNATURE ACCEPTING PATIENT

Figure 7.1. Completed patient report.

Figure 7.2. Completed patient report.

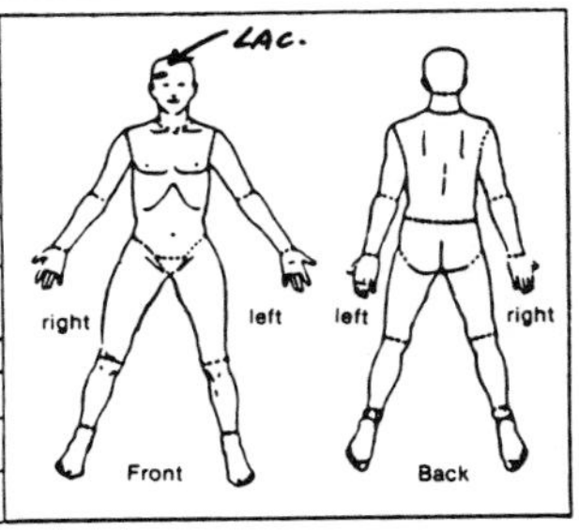

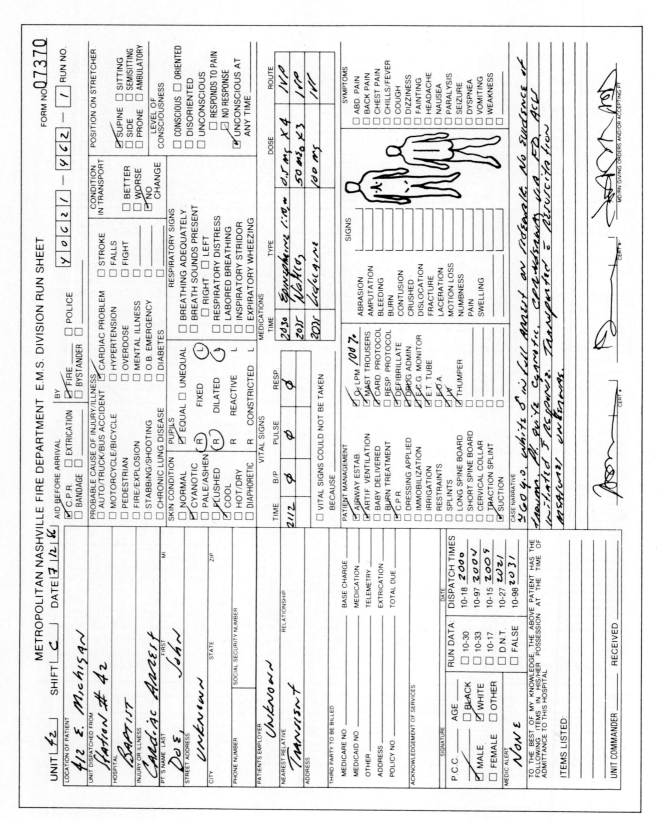

Figure 7.3. Completed patient report.

NEBRASKA EMS PATIENT ENCOUNTER FORM   **121868**

DISPATCH NO. _742_   PATIENT CONTROL NO. _421_

AGE _37_   SEX _M_   RACE ☑W ☐B ☐I ☐SS ☐OTHER   CODE _3_   ☐QRT ☐BLS ☐EMT-D ☑ALS

HISTORY

REASON FOR DISPATCH/CHIEF COMPLAINT: _Gun shot Wound to Abdomen._

CURRENT MEDICATIONS: ☑NONE

MEDICATION ALLERGIES: ☑NONE

ASSESSMENT

MENTAL STATE	PUPILS ☑Equal	SKIN ☐Normal	CHEST ☑Clear	ABDOMEN ☐Normal
☐Alert	R _____ L	☐Pale	R _____ L	☑Tender
☑Oriented	☐Reactive ☐	☐Cyanotic	☐Rales ☐	☐RUQ ☐LUQ
☐Disoriented	☐Nonreactive ☐	☐Sweaty	☐Wheezes ☐	☐RLQ ☐LLQ
☐Confused	☐Fixed ☐	☐Hot	☐Decreased ☐	☑Rigid
☐Vocal Stimulation	☐Dilated ☐	☐Cool	☐Absent ☐	☑Distended
☐Painful Stimulation	☐Constricted ☐			
☐Unresponsive				

COMMENTS: _.38 cal GSW @ upper Abdominal quadrant. Occurred 10 minutes prior to arrival._

☐TRAUMA SCORE _____ ☐CRAMS ☐SEVERITY
☐VEHICULAR _____
☑NON-VEHICULAR _____
☐MEDICAL _____
☐CARDIAC ARREST
ESTIMATED MINS DOWN PRIOR TO CPR _____

37 y.o. white ♂ c̄ .38 cal GSW to @ upper Abdomen. Splenic involvement likely. Shock.

TIME	PULSE	BP	RESP	LEVEL CONSC	RHYTHM	TREATMENT / IV / MEDICATIONS	EMT
720	120	10/60	20	(A)V P U	NSR	IV LR x 2	B.D
728	130	70/60	20	(B)V P U	NSR		
/				A V P U			
/				A V P U			
/				A V P U			

☐SEE SUPPLEMENTAL FORM

TREATMENT

AIRWAY/VENTILATION		SPLINTS	WOUND CARE	OTHER
☐Mouth to Mouth	☐CPR	☐Board	☑Dry Sterile Dressing	☑Shock Trousers
☐Oropharyngeal	☐Thumper/HLR	☐Leg Air Short	☐Wet Dressing	☐Extrication _____
☐Bag Mask	☐Bystander CPR	☐Leg Air Long	☐Occlusive Dressing	☐Restraints
☐Demand Valve	☐Defibrillation	☐Ankle Air	☐Direct Pressure	☐Reassurance
☐Esophageal Airway	**IMMOBILIZATION**	☐Arm Air	☐Pressure Dressing	☐ _____
☐Endotracheal Tube	☐Cervical Collar	☐Traction	☐Tourniquet	☐ _____
☑Oxygen _10_ LPM	☐Sandbags	☐ _____	☐ _____	☐ _____
☑Mask ☐Cannula	☐Short Spine Board	☐ _____	☐ _____	☐ _____
☐Suction	☑Long Spine Board			
☐Clear Obstructed Airway	☐			

ADMINISTRATIVE

Run Date	MO _7_ / DAY _21_ / YR _86_

		Patient's Name _Robert Brown_	Date of Birth MO _4_ / DAY _20_ / YR _48_
Time Call Received	0 7 1 5	Patient's Address _1412 S. Carter_	
Time Unit Dispatched	0 7 1 6	Pickup Location _Mel's Bar_	
Time Unit Enroute	0 7 1 6	Receiving Hospital _University_ Jones RECEIVING PHYSICIAN	Responding Service Name
1st RESPONDER ARRIVAL	0 7 1 6	Family Physician _None_	
Arrive Scene	0 7 2 0	Base Hospital _University_ BASE PHYSICIAN	Emergency Vehicle No. _714_
Depart Scene	0 7 3 5	Signatures _____	
Arrive Destination	0 7 5 0		☐VHF ☑UHF ☐LAND
Return to Service	0 8 1 5	Attendant ID's _1 4_	
Arrive Back at Station	0 8 3 0	Attendant ID's _7 2_	

SERVICE PROGRAM USE

PICK UP LOCATION
☐Street/Highway
☐Home
☐Business/Industry
☐Public Place
☑Recreation
☐Hospital
☐Nursing Home
☐ _____
Fire Zone _____
Census Tract _____
Trip Miles _____
Other Assistance By:
☑Fire Dept. ☐MD/Nurse
☑Law Enf. ☐Bystander

Dry Run
☐Care not required
☐Pt. refused care
☐Unable to locate
☐Cancelled by:

Transfer
☐Routine ☑Emergency
☐Standby
☐Fire alarm
☐ _____
☐Insurance
☐ _____
☐ _____

I have been offered and refuse
☐care ☐transportation

Signature _____

Witness _____

EMERGENCY DEPT. USE

Prehospital problems   ☐Assessment accuracy   ☐Communication
☐Treatment   ☐Timeliness
☐Request This Call Be Reviewed Locally
COMMENTS: _Excellent_

DIAGNOSIS
1. _GSW Abdomen_
2. _NIDDM_
3. _ETOH Abuse_
4.

DISPOSITION:
☐D.O.A.   ☐Admitted Acute Care   ☐Discharged – Home   ☐Discharged – Police
☐Exp in E/D   ☑Admitted, Taken to O.R. ☐Discharged – Clinic F/U ☐Transferred _____
☐Admitted – ICU, CCU ☐Admitted Observation ☐Discharged – Prv M.D. F/U ☐Other

Figure 7.4. Completed patient report.

Date	7	21	86		NEBRASKA	PAGE #	
	MO	DAY	YR		EMS PATIENT ENCOUNTER FORM SUPPLEMENT		

RESCUE SERVICE: _____   SQUAD: _____714_____   PATIENT CONTROL # 421

TIME	PULSE	BP	RESP	LEVEL CONSC	RHYTHM	TREATMENT / IV / MEDICATIONS	EMT
721	120	80/60	20	(A) V P U	Tachy cond	Lactated Ringer's	B B
722	130	70/60	20	(A) V P U	"	Lactated Ringer's	B B
				A V P U			
				A V P U			
				A V P U			
				A V P U			
				A V P U			
				A V P U			
				A V P U			
				A V P U			
				A V P U			
				A V P U			
				A V P U			
				A V P U			
				A V P U			
				A V P U			
				A V P U			
				A V P U			
				A V P U			
				A V P U			
				A V P U			
				A V P U			
				A V P U			
				A V P U			
				A V P U			
				A V P U			

COMMENTS: _____

_____

_____

_____

_____

_____

Signatures _____

Attendant ID's   [1,4] [ ] [ ]

[72] [ ] [ ]

100783

Figure 7.5. Completed patient report.

Common Abbreviations Used in EMS

ABBREVIATION	MEANING
$\bar{a}$	before
ACh	acetylcholine
ACLS	advanced cardiac life support
ALS	advanced life support
amp	ampule
α	alpha
ASA	aspirin
b.i.d.	two times a day
BLS	basic life support
β	beta
$\bar{c}$	with
c/o	complains of
Ca^{++}	calcium ion
$CaCl_2$	calcium choride
caps	capsules
cc	cublic centimeter
CHF	congestive heart failure
Cl^-	chlorine ion
cm	centimeter
cm^3	cubic centimeter
CO	carbon monoxide
COPD	chronic obstructive pulmonary disease
CSM	carotid sinus massage
CVA	cerebrovascular accident
CO_2	carbon dioxide
D/C	discontinue
dig	digitalis
DO	doctor of osteopathic medicine
Dx	diagnosis
D_5W	5% dextrose in water
$D_{50}W$	50% dextrose
EKG	electrocardiogram
elix.	elixer
EOA	esophageal obturator airway
et	and
ET	endotracheal tube
ETOH	ethyl alcohol
°F	Fahrenheit
gm	gram
gr	grain
gtts	drops
GYN	gynecological
IC	intracardiac
IM	intramuscular
IV	intravenous
K^+	potassium ion
kg	kilogram

KO	keep open
KVO	keep vein open
l	liter
lb.	pound
LBBB	left bundle branch block
LR	lactated Ringer's
MD	doctor of medicine
mEq	milliequivalents
mg	milligram
min	minute
ml	milliliter
mm	millimeter
MS	morphine sulfate
NA$^+$	sodium ion
NaHCO$_3$	sodium bicarbonate
nitro	nitroglycerin
NKA	no known allergies
non rep.	not to be repeated
NTG	nitroglycerin
N$_2$O	nitrous oxide
OB	obstetric
OD	overdose
μg	microgram
μm	micrometer
OPP	organophosphate poisoning
oz.	ounce
O$_2$	oxygen
p̄	after
PAC	premature atrial contraction
PAT	paroxysmal atrial tachycardia
pedi	pediatric
PJC	premature junctional contraction
po	by mouth
pr	per rectum
prn	as needed
PSVT	paroxysmal supraventricular tachycardia
PVC	premature ventricular contraction
q̄	every
q.h.	every hour
q.i.d.	four times a day
qt.	quart
RBBB	right bundle branch block
RL	Ringer's lactate
Rx	treatment
s̄	without
SC	subcutaneous
Sig.	let it be labeled
SL	sublingual
sol.	solution

stat	immediately
sub q	subcutaneous
t.i.d.	three times a day
TKO	to keep open
TT	transtracheal
u.	unit
ut dict.	as directed

(From Bryan Bledsoe, Gideon Bosker, and Frank Papa, *Prehospital Emergency Pharmacology*, (Bowie, Md: Brady Communications Company, Prentice-Hall, Inc., 1984), pp. 10–12.)

Bibliography

American Heart Association: "Textbook of Advanced Cardiac Life Support"; American Heart Association, Dallas, Texas, 1986

Butman A et al.: "Advanced Skills in Emergency Care: A Text For the Intermediate EMT"; Emergency Training Institute, Westport, Connecticut, 1982

Bledsoe B, Bosker G, and Papa F: "Prehospital Emergency Pharmacology"; Brady Communications Company, Bowie, Maryland, 1984

Caroline N: "Emergency Care in the Streets, 2nd Ed."; Little, Brown and Company, Boston, Massachusetts, 1983

Cohen S: "Pediatric Emergency Management": Brady Communications Company, Bowie, Maryland, 1982

Froelich R and Bishop F: "Clinical Interviewing Skills, 3rd Ed."; The C.V. Mosby Company, Saint Louis, Missouri, 1977

Gazzaniga A, Iseri L, and Baren M: "Emergency Care: Principles and Practices for the EMT-Paramedic, 2nd Ed."; Reston Publishing Company, Inc., Reston, Virginia, 1982

Guyton A: "Textbook of Medical Physiology, 6th Ed."; W.B. Saunders Company, Philadelphia, Pennsylvania, 1981

Grant H, Murray R, and Bergeron D: "Emergency Care, 4th Ed."; Brady Communications Company, Bowie, Maryland, 1986

Huszar R: "Emergency Cardiac Care, 2nd Ed."; Brady Communications Company, Bowie, Maryland 1982

Jensen S: "Paramedic Handbook"; Multi-Media Publishing Company, Denver, Colorado, 1983

Langfitt D: "Critical Care: Certification Preparation and Review"; Brady Communications Company, Bowie, Maryland, 1984

Lanros N: "Assessment and Intervention in Emergency Nursing, 2nd Ed."; Brady Communications Company, Bowie, Maryland, 1983

Malasanos L et al.: "Health Assessment, 2nd Ed."; The C.V. Mosby Company, Saint Louis, Missouri, 1981

Meltzer L, Pinneo R, and Kitchell J: "Intensive Coronary Care: A Manual for Nurses, 4th Ed."; Brady Communications Company, Bowie, Maryland, 1983

Pansky B: "Review of Gross Anatomy, 4th Ed."; Macmillan Publishing Company, Inc., New York, New York, 1979

Phillips C: "Paramedic Skills Manual"; Brady Communications Company, Bowie, Maryland, 1980

Rosen P and Sternbach G: "Atlas of Emergency Medicine, 2nd Ed."; Williams and Wilkins, Baltimore, Maryland, 1983

Rudy E and Gray V: "Handbook of Health Assessment"; Brady Communications Company, Bowie, Maryland 1981

Safer P: "Cardiopulmonary Cerebral Resuscitation"; W.B. Saunders Company, Philadelphia, Pennsylvania, 1981

Walraven G: "Basic Arrhythmias"; Brady Communications Company, Bowie, Maryland, 1980

Walraven G et al.: "Manual of Advanced Prehospital Care, 2nd Ed."; Brady Communications Company, Bowie, Maryland 1984

Glossary

Abduction: Movement away from the midline of the body.

Accessory muscles: Those muscles not normally used in respiration. However, they can be used under extreme conditions such as chronic emphysema.

Acidosis: An excess of acid in the blood (decreased pH).

Acute: Of sudden or rapid onset.

Adduction: Movement toward the midline of the body.

Afebrile: Without fever.

Affect: The inner mood or feeling.

Afferent: Carrying to the center from the periphery.

Ageusia: The loss of the sensation of taste or the ability to discriminate between various tastes (such as, sweet, sour, salty, or bitter).

Agonal: Pertaining to the period of dying.

Alkalosis: An excess of base in the blood (increased pH).

Amenorrhea: Absence of menstruation.

Analgesia: Loss of sensation, often used to describe the relief of pain without a loss of consciousness.

Anasarca: Severe, generalized body edema.

Anesthesia: The loss of sensation in an area of the body.

Aneurysm: Dilation of an artery.

Anion: An ion that carries a negative charge and, thus, is attracted to the positively charged ions (cations).

Aniscoria: Inequality of the pupils.

Anoxia: Lack of oxygen at the tissue level.

Antecubital fossa: The anterior aspect of the elbow.

Anterior: Toward the front of the body.

Anuria: Absence of excretion of urine.

Anorexia: Loss of apetite.

Aphasia: To lose the ability to express thoughts through speech.

Apical: Pertaining to the apex of the heart.

Arm: The portion of the extremity from the shoulder to the elbow.

Arrhythmia: A disturbance in the rhythm of the heart, more correctly called dysrhythmia.

Arteriosclerosis: Hardening and thickening of the walls of the arteries.

Arthritis: The inflammation of a joint.

Ascites: The accumulation of fluid in the abdomen.

Asthenia: Weakness; the loss of strength or energy.

Ataxia: Impairment of coordination of muscle activity.

Atelectasis: Collapse of the alveolar air sacs or incomplete expansion of the lung.

Atherosclerosis: The accumulation of plaques on the inner lining of the arteries.

Auscultation: The act of listening for sounds within the body.

Autotransfusion: A transfusion effected by forcing the blood from one area of the body, such as the lower extremities, to another portion of the body.

Babinski's reflex: Dorsiflexion of the great toe and fanning of the other toes following stroking of the bottom of the foot. Associated with lesions of the pyrmidal tract or motor nerves.

Battle's sign: Discoloration of the mastoid region associated with basilar skull fractures.

Borborygmus: Audible bowel sounds.

Blanch: To whiten or lighten.

Blood gases: Those gases normally found dissolved in the blood, most commonly oxygen and carbon dioxide.

Blood pressure: Pressure on the walls of the arteries created by the pumping action of the heart. Blood pressure is often a good indicator of the quality of perfusion.

Bradycardia: Heart rate less than 60 in an adult.

Bronchitis: Inflammation of one or more bronchi.

Bruit: Murmur (blowing sound) heard over peripheral blood vessels.

Buccal: Pertaining to the cheek.

Cardiac tamponade: The accumulation of blood or other fluid in the pericardial sac of such a quantity that it compresses the heart and adversely affects cardiac function.

Cardiogenic: Originating in the heart.

Cation: Positively charged ion.

Caudad: Toward the foot of the body.

Chronic obstructive pulmonary disease (COPD): A group of airway diseases that cause an obstruction to the flow of air including chronic bronchitis, emphysema, and asthma.

Clonus: Rhythmic alteration between contraction or relaxation of muscles induced by stretching the muscle.

Colloid: A solution containing a protein such as albumin.

Coma: Deep unconsciousness from which a patient cannot be aroused.

Consensual: Reflex action in one pupil mimicking that occurring in the other pupil.

Contralateral: On the opposite side of the body.

Cor pulmonale: Disease of the heart secondary to diseases of the lungs.

Craniad: Toward the head.

Crepitation: A dry crackling sound associated with: subcutaneous emphysema, fractures, and dry synovial joints.

Crystalloid: A solution that contains only electrolytes or carbohydrates.

Cyanosis: Dark, bluish discoloration of the skin and mucous membranes

associated with a decreased delivery of oxygen to the tissues.

Deja vu: A sensation that you have "been there before."

Diplopia: Double vision.

Disorientation: Lack of awareness to either person, place, or time.

Dysmenorrhea: Painful menstruation.

Dysphagia: Difficult or painful swallowing.

Dyspnea: Difficult or labored breathing.

Dysuria: Difficult or painful urination.

Eccymosis: A bluish discoloration (bruising) of the skin resulting from intradermal or submucosal hemorrhage.

Ectopic: Abnormally located.

Edema: An abnormal increase in the amount of interstitial fluid in a given region or area of the body.

Efferent: Carrying from the center to the periphery.

Embolism: The movement of a clot or of a foreign substance through a blood vessel.

Emphysema: The accumulation of air in tissues or organs.

Emesis: Vomiting.

Encephalitis: Inflammation of the brain.

Epiphora: Abnormal tearing of the eyes.

Epistaxis: Hemorrhage from the nose, often associated with a blow to the nose or, occasionally, hypertension.

Erythema: The enlargment of the capillaries causing redness of the skin.

Fever: Elevation of body temperature above that considered normal for an individual. Fever indicates a resetting of the body's temperature set point and should not be confused with hyperthermia.

Flaccid: Without tone, flabby.

Forearm: The portion of the upper extremity distal to the elbow.

Fremitus: Palpable vibration.

Friction rub: A crackling, grating sound heard through the stethoscope when two inflamed surfaces, such as the pleura, rub together.

Gallop rhythm: Heart rate characterized by three sounds in the presence of a tachycardia.

Goiter: Increase in the size of the thyroid gland.

Hematemesis: Vomiting of blood.

Hematoma: The localized collection of blood associated with rupture of a blood vessel.

Hematuria: The presence of blood in the urine.

Hemoptysis: The coughing up of blood.

Hypertension: The persistent elevation of the blood pressure.

Hypertrophy: The increase in the size of a tissue or organ.

Hypoglossal: Below the tongue.

Infarction: Obstruction of the circulation followed by tissue necrosis.

Ipsilateral: On the same side.

Keratitis: Inflammation of the cornea.

Menorrhagia: Excessive menstruation.

Migraine: Headaches, often severe, associated with dilation of blood vessels of the brain. Migraine is often unilateral and occasionally preceded by an aura.

Murmur: Blowing sound caused by turbulent blood flow.

Mydriasis: Extreme dilatation of the pupils, often associated with oculomotor nerve paralysis.

Nausea: Feeling that emesis is impending.

Neuralgia: Pain associated with the course of a nerve.

Nuchal: Pertaining to the nape (back) of the neck.

Nystagmus: Involuntary, rhythmic movements of the eyes in any plane.

Oliguria: Abnormally decreased production of urine.

Orthopnea: The inability to breathe while lying in the supine position.

Palpate: To examine by touching.

Palpitation: A patient's awareness of the, often rapid, pulses.

Papilledema: Edema of the optic papilla. Often associated with hypertension.

Paraesthesia: Abnormal sensory sensations which may include burning, itching, or the feeling of electrical shocks.

Percussion: Examination conducted by listening to reverberation after striking the surface with short, sharp blows.

Peristalsis: Wave of contraction that moves material through the gastrointestinal tract.

Photophobia: Abnormal visual intolerance to light.

Pleural effusion: Fluid of any kind in the pleural cavity.

Pleurisy: Pain accompanying pleural inflammation.

Priapism: Prolonged erection of the penis.

Pulse: Palpable rhythmic expansion of an artery.

Pyrexia: Fever.

Rale: Breath sound that sounds like fine crackling because of the movement of air through an exudate.

Rhonchi: Coarse, rattling sounds, somewhat like snoring, usually because of secretions in the bronchi.

Stereognosis: Discrimination of objects by the sense of touch.

Stridor: Harsh, high-pitched respiratory sound associated with severe upper airway obstruction.

Symptom: An abnormal feeling of distress and/or awareness of disturbance of bodily function experienced by a patient.

Syncope: Fainting, temporary unconsciousness.

Syndrome: Consistent group of signs and symptoms that are produced by a similar pathological change in different individuals.

Tachycardia: Heart rate greater than 100 beats per minute in an adult.

Tachypnea: Rapid respiratory rate.

Thrill: Palpable murmur; vibration accompanying turbulence in the heart or great vessels.

Tremor: An involuntary twitching of an extremity.

Trimester: A period of 13 weeks.

Ulcer: An open lesion on the skin or mucous membrane.

Urticaria: Hives.

Vagus: The tenth cranial nerve.

Vertex: The top of the head.

Vertigo: Dizziness, a sense that the external world is spinning around.

Vital signs: Measurements of body functions including pulse, respirations, blood pressure, and temperature.

Zygoma: The cheek bone.

Index